A Frenchwoman's Guide to
SEX AFTER SIXTY

• • •

MARIE DE HENNEZEL

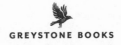

GREYSTONE BOOKS

Vancouver/Berkeley

Greystone Books Ltd.
www.greystonebooks.com

Cataloguing data available from Library and Archives Canada
ISBN 978-1-77164-334-4 pbk
ISBN 978-1-77164-335-1 ePub

Cover and text design by Nayeli Jimenez
Typesetting by Shed Simas/Onça Design
Cover photograph by Randy Faris/Corbis/VCG
Printed and bound in Canada on ancient-forest-friendly paper by Friesens

We gratefully acknowledge the support of the Canada Council for the Arts, the British
Columbia Arts Council, the Province of British Columbia through the Book Publishing Tax
Credit, and the Government of Canada for our publishing activities.

Canada

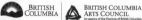

BRITISH
COLUMBIA

BRITISH COLUMBIA
ARTS COUNCIL
An agency of the Province of British Columbia

Canada Council   Conseil des arts
for the Arts   du Canada

Mantra for *Sex After Sixty*

* * *

When we are lovers of love,
we remain so all our lives.
There is no age limit for loving desire,
erotic joy, or physical intimacy.
We just need to let our hearts and bodies
do their thing; they know how to make love.
If we try to recreate what we experienced
at a younger age, there'll be no hope for us.

CONTENTS

. . .

INTRODUCTION

• • •

A future for loving intimacy

WHEN MY BOOK *The Warmth of the Heart Prevents Your Body from Rusting* was first published in English, readers reacted to one chapter in particular: "A Sensual Old Age," which focuses on the sexuality of seniors, a subject that still remains taboo. At the suggestion of my editor, I decided to dedicate an entire book to that topic. I wanted to understand the ways my perspective as a Frenchwoman could interest foreign readers, so I started to research. While digging into various publications regarding sexuality over age 60, I was struck by a particularly American obsession with youth. The focus for North American women seems to be on working out at the gym and undergoing cosmetic surgery to stay young and sexy looking as they advance in years. The standard of youth as the norm is also reflected in their approach to sexuality and seduction as they age.

I wanted to show that if there's no age limit to enjoying love, if making love is still an option, that is because *the heart does not age*, not because the body works to remain young. The body will age, sooner or later, but if we create intimacy in everyday life, develop our sensuality, and let tenderness bring our bodies together, then we can live out what I call a different kind of sexuality for a very long time. And in my experience, as well as that of the many men and women I've met these past few years, it is just as satisfying.

In fact, I am pleading for *a new sexual revolution*—one for seniors. I have realized, after many conversations, that though we acknowledge that making love at age 70 will not be the same as at age 30, our generation has no desire to renounce sex; we are ready to invent something new. Is this specifically French?

"I am pleading for *a new sexual revolution*—one for seniors."

I belong to the generation that led the "sexual revolution" of the 1970s in France. We broke down many barriers and we fought for the rights to contraception and abortion. We are not afraid to fight the youth-obsessed culture that is hindering the sexuality of seniors. The goal is not to preserve the bodies we had when we were young but rather to maintain our health, ourselves, and our desires so that our bodies age as well as possible. Ours is a dynamic generation, generous and selfish at once, driven by the urge to travel, learn, and explore new territory. In short, a generation that has desires.

This book is written for them and for anyone turning 60: men and women who may already have noticed their bodies start to age sexually and may be wondering what the future holds for their sex lives. For the most part, they still have over a third of their lives ahead. How will they experience their later years? With or without sex?

A recent study published by the Korian Institute for Ageing Well on the relationship between age and pleasure reveals that while only 12 percent of people over the age of 65 find that making love is still a source of pleasure, 36 percent of them would like it to be.[1] This means there is quite a significant gap between those who would like to be sexually active at this age and those who continue to be and find it pleasurable.

So there are clearly obstacles to sexual fulfilment beyond a certain age. Some are related to circumstances, aloneness, and the attitude of our youth-obsessed society. But others stem from the image people have of themselves, of their bodies—seen as desirable or not—and the importance they give to Eros, sexual pleasure, both in their lives in general and in their specific relationships. The ultimate obstacle is the difficulty of imagining a different kind of sexuality, one that is less impulsive, slower and more sensual; one that puts connectedness, tenderness, and intimacy first.

However, the research I conducted for over a year proves that there is no age limit to love, sex, and desire, even if we hide it after a certain age. It is like an intimate secret that we don't want to reveal but that plays a key role in the physical and psychological health of older people. As people believed in ancient China, loving sex leads to a long and happy life. Some even say that with age, "sex is better, lasts longer and is more erotic,"[2] because older women are thought to give themselves more intensely and to offer their bodies and souls more fully.

> "There is no age limit to love, sex, and desire,
> even if we hide it after a certain age."

Does this pursuit of sexual activity relate to our character, to a predisposition to love that we have always had and continue to have? Undoubtedly. And we could leave it at that. Tell ourselves that if we were keen on sex before, we always will be. That it's not worth writing a whole book about it. But the reality is more complex.

For example, what makes so many sexagenarians who find themselves alone in life look for their soulmate on internet dating sites, in the rather elusive quest for the perfect partner? Once they retire, some people seem to take advantage of their newfound freedom to relive their youth and enjoy a level of sensuality they may not have experienced when they were younger.

What is this creative attitude towards sexuality that compels people to change the way they love and explore new sensual pleasures—women by giving themselves more fully, men by being slower and gentler, couples by probing the hidden depths of their intimacy? This book will discuss everything older adults can learn from Eastern erotic arts such as Tantra and Taoism.

Finally, what drives sexual attraction in older men and women? Modern society is so youth oriented that it's hard for us to imagine sex between two ageing bodies. So what is this desire that isn't fueled by appearance or physical beauty but by something else—by someone's charm, intense gaze, bright smile? What is this desire that stems from the pleasure and excitement of being together—two hearts beating as one, touching each other's skin, and feeling each other's movements and presence—even very late in life?

These are the questions I have asked throughout my research on sexuality and 60-somethings. I have come to one sure-fire conclusion: the erotic intimacy many want, but few achieve, requires a complete change in mindset. Experts agree that we can't make love at 60 like we did at 40. Our bodies can't keep up. So we must let go of what we know, forget about sexual performance and old fantasies, and "let love happen." In other words, we must learn to take pleasure as it comes rather than focus on what it should be. The quality of the relationship is key, along with the ability to create intimacy in everyday life. Many people think this kind of sex—which is less focused on genitalia and more erotic—is in fact an improvement.

By writing this book, I hope to make people look at the future of our sexual intimacy in a different way. I know many older people would love to experience this new sexuality, which the philosopher Robert Misrahi says could "contribute to enhancing old age." I'm thinking in particular of those who are lucky enough to still be in a relationship but who no longer have the energy for sex.[3]

"The erotic intimacy that many want, but few
achieve, requires a complete change in mindset."

I also have in mind passionate older women, who may be alone because they are widowed or separated but who dream of meeting someone new, and the ageing men who would like to keep having sex but who are scared of not seeming virile enough and being rejected because of it, those who are tempted to turn to younger women so they can feel young again, and those who want to try changing their sex life within an existing relationship.

Finally, I hope to encourage our children's and grand-children's generations to look more sympathetically on loving in old age so that they learn to treat it with respect and kindness.

This book does not pretend to cover all aspects of this question. It is not an exhaustive study. It is more like a diary of sorts, in which I aim to strike a balance between modesty and immodesty, as I write about the mystery and depth of ageing people's love lives. I invite readers to follow me on my journey as I research this unexplored subject through my meetings with people, the books and articles I read, and my own thinking on the matter, as well as my detours to the distant realms of Tantra and other Eastern erotic arts.

• • •

CHAPTER ONE

The age of pleasure and desire

Is it possible to maintain an erotic love life after 60?
If so, what must one do? What changes are necessary?

• • •

A T THE TIME I began writing this book, an exhibition
about the *Kamasutra*, subtitled "Spirituality and
Eroticism in Indian Art," was being held at the Pina-
cothèque Gallery in Paris.[4]

It is worth pointing out to Westerners who might
think the *Kamasutra* is just a pornographic book, a
treatise on erotic acrobatics and a collection of sexual
positions, that it is a very ancient "book of life" address-
ing the role of sexuality in helping men and women lead
a fulfilled life. Its purpose is to show that to live happily,
we need balance between *dharma*, which means virtue;
artha, material prosperity; and *kama*, love and pleasure.
According to Hindu beliefs, living your life with a focus
on eroticism—putting pleasure at the center of everything
you do and experience—leads to *moksha*, or liberation, and
spiritual awakening.

Eroticism represents a path to fulfilment and to the
divine. On the information panel at the entrance to the
exhibition was written: "If in Christianity God *is* love, in
India God *makes* love."[5] Followed further on by: "Love is
not an affair of the heart but of the body."

As I wandered through the engravings and statues, I realized I was at the core of a radically different mindset from ours in the West. Many Indian religions state that to achieve liberation and wisdom, a form of asceticism is needed. Here, we believe the opposite. There, humans who have achieved their quest for pleasure can finally be liberated—because you can only be set free from what you have experienced fully. Like the fruit that falls off the tree when it's ripe. In India, the third age is the age of maturity, and this age has a duty to fully experience the state of *kama*, loving desire and pleasure.

If we remain focused on performance-based sex, we're done for!

IS THE THIRD age really, as was stated in ancient India, the age of loving pleasure and desire? I consider the following paradox: on the one hand, we are told that sexuality is a human right, regardless of age, that maintaining a sex life is the secret to longevity and good health, that the belief that sexuality is synonymous with youth is completely wrong, as a large percentage of older people are sexually active and still have desires; on the other hand, we read that sexual ageing does take place and our libido decreases with age. What is the reality?

I decide to discuss the question with several experts in France, particularly with my dear friend François Parpaix, a sex therapist I have known for a long time, and then Brigitte Lahaie, because she is, in my view, an authority on the sex lives of the French. The answers are clear: we have to be realistic when we talk about sexual pleasure and desire in older adults. We have to face the facts: of course sexual ageing takes place. The senses become dulled, arousal is slow, hormonal changes lead to decreased desire, reactions are less intense, men suffer from erectile dysfunction,[6] getting less hard, for less time and less often, women develop vaginal dryness and atrophy, except if they are on hormone replacement therapy (HRT), getting wet less often and more slowly. It takes longer and longer to reach orgasm. Making love can become tiring and uncomfortable because our mobility and flexibility decrease and we suffer from rheumatism and pains. Our figures change, our muscles waste, and we put on weight. All of this affects our body image. We see ourselves as old in other people's eyes and therefore as less desirable. And then there are all the medicines, antidepressants, diuretics, and mood-enhancing psychotropic drugs, as well as the treatments for diabetes: they impact our sex lives and libidos. Two-thirds of older adults believe that their ability to make love will diminish over the next decade.

I'm stunned by the depressing picture my research paints. It seems to confirm the belief that is deeply rooted in our personal and collective unconscious: *sex is for young people*. Most older adults see it in the same way: sexuality in an elderly person goes against the grain; it's ridiculous and inappropriate. When we're old, we can no longer become aroused or feel desire.

I pursue my research well aware that I shouldn't be naively optimistic about sexuality for the older generation. That said, despite sexual ageing, people do nonetheless have erotic love lives well beyond the age of 60,[7] especially those who enjoyed making love when they were young, and if they are still in a relationship.

But there is one condition: we cannot focus on *sexual performance*. Older adults who were used to orgasm- and ejaculation-based sex soon find themselves backed into a corner with no room for maneuver. As long as our body is functioning physiologically, we aren't let down. But as soon as our physiology deteriorates, sexual organs lose their ability to get wet or hard or to ejaculate. When we find it difficult to get into a position because it hurts our backs or hips, when we lose our breath, or when a woman can no longer bear her partner's weight, we can't rely on our bodies anymore. And that can completely put people off making love.

Developing erotic skills

CONSEQUENTLY, WE HAVE to start developing something else: the ability to be erotic, to seduce, and to let ourselves be kissed and caressed.

Maintaining an erotic love life beyond the age of 60 requires a *brand-new approach* to sex: less focus on genitalia and more on being erotic. The quality of the relationship is obviously key, as is taking our time, letting our partner take theirs, exploring slower-paced and more sensual, tender, and playful sex, in which emotions and intimacy play a leading role, and being able to take pleasure as it comes and not focus on *what it should be*. It is no less satisfying an experience. Far from it.

Of course if we stay fixated on the idea of impulsive sex and compare ourselves with what we experienced when we were 40, we'll tell ourselves it's not as good. That's why we have to change our tune.

Yet not everyone can make this shift. Many older people prefer to draw a line through their sex lives, because sex basically doesn't interest them that much, and the time has come to turn the page. But others will take advantage of waving goodbye to "performance-based sex," because sex has always been important to them. They still know how to seduce each other, and thanks to that eroticism they have never let their sexuality stagnate. They have an erotic understanding that dates from their earliest youth, no doubt.

Creating intimacy in everyday life

I ASK MY friend François Parpaix about his older patients. It turns out that older people mainly consult with him when they're embarking on a new romance following widowhood or separation. "It's mostly women who bring their partners. The man plays down his erection problem, even though it bothers him a great deal, while the woman expects something more from their relationship. Thanks to my experience as a sex therapist, I can deduce that the real reason for the consultation is issues surrounding *intimacy*."

Again, one must distinguish physiological sensations (which can't be as intense at the age of 60 as they were at 40, since they diminish with age) and the perception of pleasure, which encompasses the emotional quality of the relationship.

This is why, according to François, some women say they have much better orgasms after the age of 60. The love, intimate connectedness, and emotional imagination involved in the erotic encounter give them the impression of climaxing like they never have before. "These women," François adds, "often don't need the man's erection in order to come."[8] They need an emotional environment with caresses and deep, languorous kisses. They have an erotic imagination and can focus on their perineum and lose themselves in pleasure. François shares the example of a 75-year-old female patient of his who recently told him, "I don't really give a damn that my husband doesn't get hard anymore. Even without the goods, he still makes me come."

"One must distinguish physiological sensations (which can't be as intense at the age of 60 as they were at 40, since they diminish with age) and the perception of pleasure, which encompasses the emotional quality of the relationship."

But men have trouble understanding that. "For them, getting a hard-on is very important. It's part of their masculine identity," he says, and tells me about a visit from a 94-year-old man who arrived at his practice by taxi, walking stick in hand, and told him, "I'm in love with a 75-year-old woman. When I lie down with her, I can't get an erection anymore. I lost my wife 15 years ago and haven't made love since. Give me some Viagra." François prescribed him some but explained that the woman might be hoping for something else.

François and I agree: ageing couples face the challenge of keeping that loving feeling—or else tenderness and companionship—alive by creating moments of intimacy throughout the day.

The art of reaching out and understanding each other, being comfortable with your masculinity or femininity, remaining attractive to your partner, keeping your sense of humor, being imaginative and sensual, are all things that have to be learned. Seduction has to be learned. So François gives his patients various tips.

For instance, to create erotic intimacy, he suggests establishing a ritual to bring out each other's sexual energy: look into each other's eyes for one minute every day, wrap your arms around one another, heart chakra to heart chakra, groin to groin, and breathe in unison for 20 seconds every day. That will stimulate desire. The couple enters into a sort of erotic "dance" that François refers to as the "intimate, erotic in-between": the art of sexually arousing each other in purposeful little steps, neither too fast nor too slow, from foreplay to a sensual, erotic union that may or may not include orgasm and ejaculation. This type of sensual pleasure holds an important place in older people's lives and often replaces sexual intercourse. It is an erotic art, without constraints or rules, in which people have the right to fail, regardless of the means used—caresses, sex toys, positions—and which takes into account each person's experience and vulnerability.

This erotic intimacy involves giving in to desires and not worrying about image. Many people are too vain to do this erotic dance because they can't stop looking at themselves and tense up over their self-image: "I look ugly, I've got love handles, I've got cellulite, my penis is rubbish, oh when I think how shapely my bottom/breasts used to be!"

Comparing our current selves to our younger selves automatically leads to failure.

But this level of intimacy isn't relevant to all couples. Sex might no longer interest them or might have stopped working for them. "We have to stop promoting sexuality to those couples, stop hyping miracle sex until we're 90." We can experience physical closeness, companionship, and intimate connectedness without involving the sexual organs.

"Seduction has to be learned."

So François insists we consider three other "ways of making love": tenderness, empathy, and connectedness. He recommends creating a ritual of tender intimacy: gazing lovingly at one another, putting your hand on the other, moving away, moving together again, brushing lips, hugging, being next to each other. You shouldn't snuggle up in the other's arms like a child, because that means you are seeking security and protection, and this distorts matters.

In order to maintain empathy and connectedness, it's important to take the time to sit down and tell one another what you've been doing, share that day's emotions, and say how you sense the other is feeling ("You seem tense"). It's also key to show gratitude for what your partner gives you and to be able to work in harmony on joint projects.

François says that if these three levels of intimacy exist in a relationship, the partners will be happy, even if they no longer make love "genitally."

Not everyone finds it easy

FRANÇOIS AND I both greatly admire the French radio talk-show host Brigitte Lahaie, who also happens to be a movie actress and former adult film star. In her program *Lahaie, l'amour et vous* ("Lahaie, Love, and You") on RMC, listeners from every walk of life call in to share their sexual problems with her. Because Brigitte is, as her loyal French following knows, "the woman who knows, who has experienced it all, has tried (nearly) everything and to whom you can tell all." And can trust.

When I ask her if she thinks the third age is the age of pleasure and desire, her initial reaction is skeptical. "I'm 60 years old and I can tell you things were better when I was 40. I was more supple, more desirable." I remind her that in the book she wrote about a decade ago, she said there was no age limit for love, and people could "have sex till the day they die."[9] Brigitte acknowledges that it's possible, but rare.

She too refuses to promote the idea that sex is better at 60 than at 40 and explains that most women over 60 are ageing sexually. Many of them have had a truly satisfying sex life and shouldn't think it's going to improve as they get older. What's more, the older they get, the more often they find themselves on their own. And when you're on your own with rather low self-esteem and a broken heart, it's easy to slide into depression. You withdraw into yourself, you become detached and hardened. Sexuality is relegated to a distant memory. Even the idea of a fulfilling sex life seems absurd.

Brigitte has clearly witnessed frustrations and failures: men who feel inadequate; women who wonder if they make love often enough and have proper orgasms; women who are often uncomfortable with their bodies and not as liberated as we might believe despite society's changing attitudes and openness about sex; women influenced by women's magazines, which prescribe a mechanical vision of sexuality that is completely at odds with their innermost feelings—one that emphasizes the obligation to perform and therefore doesn't help them achieve a happy, fulfilling sex life.

So it is difficult to believe we can have a fulfilling sex life in older age. But when a relationship is based on loving intimacy, couples can experience *different sensual pleasure*: slower, more intense, and focused more on union than on sexual excitement.

Indeed, as discussed, sexuality in older adults can't be *the same*. But it is no less satisfying as a result. Take 66-year-old Paul, who told Brigitte Lahaie he still makes love once or twice a week. "Cuddles and tenderness now form the focus of sex with my wife. I won't claim I can perform in the same way I did 30 years ago. But even so my sex life remains very, very satisfying."

What then should we make of 75-year-old Line's story? The older she gets, "the more wonderful her sex life becomes." She has a new partner who is 66 years old, and she experiences "extraordinary orgasms" with him.[10]

These accounts echo those reported by another French sex therapist, Alain Héril.[11] In one, Mathilde, aged 68, experiences "an abundance of orgasms" and discovers she is a female ejaculator. "For the first time in her life (at over 60 years old), she feels her heart leap, is overwhelmed by an incredibly powerful desire—morning, noon, and night—and delights in re-living the excitement of her teenage years." And Rosemonde, aged 70, who says she is experiencing "the pinnacle of her desire" and loving it. She doesn't mean she hasn't experienced anything like it before, but what she's discovering with her second husband is *unexpected and magical.* "It isn't more intense," she says, "it's *more open, expansive.*"[12]

"When a relationship is based on loving intimacy, couples can experience *different sensual pleasure*: slower, more intense, and focused more on union than on sexual excitement."

Héril admits he is deeply moved each time women recount the exceptional experiences that made them cry with joy, which they'd never experienced or even imagined before. "During those moments, sexuality is characterized by *an energy based only on the beauty of pleasure* ... The result is something simple and glorious. They don't really have anything to prove to each other anymore."[13]

"But those women," retorts Brigitte Lahaie when I bring this up, "are women who have always been great lovers. They feel happy with their bodies and have established strong feminine identities. They have always loved making love and have learned how to be grounded in their sensual pleasure. They are driven by curiosity and a robust, triumphant lust for life, which encourages them to explore unknown territory. Not everyone can do that. The question is: why do some women find it easy and others don't?"

What are the obstacles?

OVER THE FOLLOWING weeks, I try to find out what is stopping physical fulfilment as we grow older.

It takes two to make love. Many women over 60 find themselves on their own because they are divorced or their partner has died. Unlike the European grandmothers of yesteryear, they no longer wear those little black ribbons (known in France as *je-ne-baise-plus*[14]) around their necks, although they may just as well. Alongside the women who are no longer interested in men and even feel relieved that they don't have to make love anymore, and those who find "the gymnastics complicated" and are very pleased to have drawn a line through their sex lives, there are all those whose feelings of desire are still very much alive. In the absence of a life partner, these women would very much like to meet a new lover. Yet they don't. Is loneliness unavoidable?

Psychoanalysts would say these women aren't ready or even clear about why they want to get their sex lives going again.

As a result, this period of loneliness, which is very common around age 60, is also a period during which we grow. It provides the opportunity for us to learn to feel good about ourselves and to enjoy our own company, to develop real autonomy, and to find out what we want to do, what we like, and what counts the most.

These days, sex therapists' consulting rooms are full of sexagenarians wanting to become "sexy-genarians." Are they victims of advertising's obsession with sexual fulfilment? Having not yet experienced sexual fulfilment, do they want to achieve it before they're over the hill? The reasons for their behavior are actually more complex. These women are baby boomers. In France, they belong to the generation that took part in the civil uprisings of May 1968. They have also lived through pseudo-sexual liberation. I say "pseudo" because talking freely about sexuality hasn't been enough to help these women achieve erotic freedom. This generation often feels today, in their *young old age*, that they've missed out on the most important aspects of erotic joy. They know that eroticism is an essential part of being human—a "sacred" dimension, a source of joy and balance. Women of my generation may have neglected it during their lives. They are vaguely aware that there is a *spiritual* dimension to meeting and physically connecting with the other, and they want to experience it before they die.

They've realized that analyzing themselves, their desires and identities as ageing women, is crucial.

How did they develop as sexual beings? Of course, the key is in each woman's personal history. And it's the first thing a sex therapist will try to understand. Were they sexually abused? Raped? A shocking number of women were interfered with when they were children, and that abuse leaves deep scars. They need to be extremely resilient if they are going to overcome their resultant fear of or disgust towards men.

Have they experienced some kind of "war of the sexes" founded on a very poor image of men—as predators, as sex maniacs, bastards "with one-track minds"? That image often derives from their fathers or the way their mothers talked about men. Or were they fortunate enough to be attracted to men from the day they were born, experiencing them as gentle, fragile, tender beings who they want to protect or seduce?

We also have to look at what was forbidden in their education or religion. This can impact how women feel about their own nudity, for example. We need to examine the intuitive image that a woman has of her mother's sexuality. It is known that a mother can unconsciously forbid or authorize her daughter to experience sexual pleasure. Did the woman develop her personality by subscribing to her mother's imagined enjoyment of sex or by rejecting it? By rebelling against her mother's nonenjoyment of sex or by supporting it? Taboos surrounding sexuality were broken down 40 years ago, and yet the majority of today's 60-somethings are still unwittingly entangled in the sexuality of other women in their families.

There comes a time when it is not too late to sort out your life and free yourself from the weight of the past. The transition into our 60s can be a good time to do so. I am always amazed to see the transformation that occurs in women who have the courage to take this step. A course of psychotherapy, however brief, helps unblock the dam of desire. It's worth giving it a go.

Once we break free from the past, are we ready for the narcissistic revolution that is essential for erotic freedom at this age?

I think back to the account of the 70-year-old woman who, during one of my talks on the art of ageing well, exclaimed: "I see nothing very sexy or physically attractive about these folds and this shriveled skin. It deteriorates with age. I don't believe at all in this naive optimism that tries to convince us that 'it gets better and better.' Let's be honest, we lose what made us happy in our 40s, 50s, and even 60s, and it's tenderness and sweet memories that enrich what sexuality remains. There is nothing exciting about growing old!"

So many women lack self-esteem and keep a constant eye out for changes in their faces. They think they look ugly, and a little voice inside their heads tells them no man will ever want them. If by chance these women do meet someone, they take one look at themselves, tense up, and shut themselves off instead of giving in to their feelings.

"There comes a time when it is not too late to sort out your life and free yourself from the weight of the past. The transition into our 60s can be a good time to do so."

To define the narcissistic revolution in question, we can think of Woody Allen's line: "I never look at myself in the mirror anymore, as it's depressing. I look inside myself because inside I'm young." The same should apply to women, of course! We have to shift our thoughts from the "body we have," the one we see in the mirror, to the "body we are," the physical body that we feel. "I don't really care about seeing my body grow older," said a girlfriend of my age. "I feel good inside." Her priority is feeling positive and taking care of herself. She has realized that the changes in her body have nothing to do with the strength of her desire. She gives more importance to being radiant than being wrinkled. She remains young in her mind, and that impacts the way she looks, carries herself, and lets herself go in bed. Like all women who feel young at heart, she looks after herself, dresses with care, wears perfume, and stays in shape through swimming and yoga. In short, she tries to look good. No need for cosmetic surgery. In his book *La Jouissance*, Jean-Luc Nancy wrote: "A woman is beautiful when she knows she is desired." We could add: "and she is desired when she has desires." Obsessing over how she looked as a young woman won't help her achieve this narcissistic revolution.

• • •

CHAPTER TWO

Second adolescence

*What is the cost of baby boomers' obsession
with youth? And what must they do to
enjoy a more fulfilling sexual life?*

• • •

The sexual boom in senior citizens

EVERY DAY WE read articles about the sexual boom in senior citizens. The phenomenon seems to fascinate journalists aged 35 to 50, because it relates to the sexuality of their parents—parents who are experiencing something completely different from what their own parents experienced at the same age. We are witnessing a shift, and we know the factors driving it: medical advances, changing attitudes, the prevalence of pleasure, and the desire to stay young for as long as possible.

The baby boomer generation, which found sexual freedom, instituted contraception, and legalized abortion, doesn't think twice about getting divorced at 60 and starting a new relationship that they hope will be more emotionally and sexually fulfilling than the previous one.[15] But this is also a fragile generation that has bought heavily into modern society's obsession with youth and is ultimately not as liberated as we think. By flaunting sex everywhere, the media have established norms that are hard to escape. There's a lot of pressure to climax. This "right to have orgasms and desires" is part of a general wish to live longer and age well.[16]

"The explosion of porn on the internet has fueled people's sexual fantasies. Some retired men spend entire days on their computers, masturbating to porn till late at night. But when they slip under the sheets, they're alone once again," says François Parpaix. "It's a similar scenario with their wives. Whereas in the past they would have twiddled their thumbs, now they're chatting on the internet. These activities are more exciting and romantic, but ultimately the act of seeking out pleasure on their own creates a lack of intimacy within the relationship that often leads to separation. However, as men hate living alone and women are always on the lookout for love, they put themselves back on the market. But once they go on dating sites, they realize how hard it is to resume their sex lives. So they come to me to ask for a little blue pill, or lubricant gel for the women."

Behind this physiological need lies a deeper problem. These people are faced with issues they thought they'd put aside. Some of them think they were bad lovers, that their sex life wasn't up to much, and they want to reignite it before it's too late. The truth is they still have a lot to learn, which is probably why sexagenarians in the throes of love appear to be going through a "second adolescence."

François affectionately calls them "sexual illiterates," with a touch of irony. They capitalize on their renewed interest in sex by reading erotic literature and watching raunchy films together. This reawakens their physical chemistry and makes them feel young again.

Although this can be a trap that shuts when their bodies are unable to keep up, it can also be an opportunity for them to invent a new approach to sexuality and sometimes even establish a second sex life. This means they have to say goodbye to the performance-based sex of their younger years and embrace the *different kind of sexuality* I spoke about at the start of this book—a sexuality that is more relational, sensual, and tender.

Rejuvenating hearts and bodies

THAT SAID, THIS second adolescence comes at a price: destroying the couple.

I recently heard the philosopher Yann Dall'Aglio[17] give a talk on "another way to love" at the Festival of Cabourg in France. As the title suggests, Dall'Aglio is interested in how the way we love is evolving. Nowadays we try to experience love within a committed relationship, and it's clearly not working. This is because in the old days, couples used to stay together not out of love, but out of duty and necessity. Today, "we want to experience the same emotional intensity within marriage that in the past could only be produced by distance and illicit affairs,"[18] he says. This can only lead to one thing: the "disintegration of relationships" and the breakdown of couples. People embark on a passionate quest for romance, governed by the standards and demands of consumerism: effectiveness, performance, and sexual enjoyment at all costs.

And when the "love and sex" columns in magazines talk about "efforts needed and the techniques to use," "it's not to give love a human dimension [...] or to convert passion into tenderness, friendship, or intimate jokes," says Dall'Aglio, but to "revive lost passion and *rejuvenate hearts and bodies* using Kamasutra-style acrobatics, clothes, and gifts. But when we see these men and women—whose worn-out bodies literally and metaphorically bear the scars of divorce and pregnancy—dressing up like teenagers, panting their lungs out on the treadmill, slathering cream on their skin, and flashing brilliant white smiles; when we hear them say they're looking for the 'love of their lives' for the third, fourth, or umpteenth time, it's impossible to believe them."[19]

"People embark on a passionate quest for romance, governed by the standards and demands of consumerism: effectiveness, performance, and sexual enjoyment at all costs."

Psychoanalyst Jean-Michel Hirt[20] has also written about the harm caused by programs about love, or series that continually order us to be happier, more in love, and more desirable, to a generation founded on a culture of self-obsession. We expect too much from marriage: perfect harmony, mutual fulfilment, cast-iron certainties. And we know how difficult it is to look away from all these mirrors.

The illusion of ideal love

"THE MYTH OF Prince Charming, of the soulmate, is ingrained in our subconscious," writes Alain Héril in a psychologies.com web chat. This myth is now affecting sexagenarians. While few of them are currently signed up to dating websites (less than 10 percent), the ones who are, are hoping to meet the love of their lives. On rare occasions, some succeed: they find their needle in a haystack. But most are disappointed and end up leaving the site.

I recently had a small group of single women to my home, all of whom are registered with Attractive World, a French dating site "for discerning singles."

Alain Héril: "The myth of Prince Charming, of the soulmate, is ingrained in our subconscious."

We talk non-stop about their experiences, discussing the range of emotions that preceded the symbolic gesture of signing up. First, the fear of risk: "What if I meet some weirdo or pervert?" And shame: "Why on Earth am I selling myself on the internet?" "This is creepy!" "It's the last thing I need!" We speak about the courage it takes to expose yourself, to admit you need love and can't stand being alone anymore. Creating your online profile is an experience in its own right. It forces you to face yourself and define who you are clearly. It's a conscious act. We find ourselves laughing quite a bit.

Flo92, a well-known former journalist, aged 69, tells us about her first date with a retired top media executive. They instantly recognized each other and burst out laughing. What were they doing on the site? They both admitted that their fame had become an obstacle. They were also surrounded by well-established couples. By concealing their identities, they felt they had a better chance of meeting single people.

Pimprenelle, a 62-year-old pharmacist with a round face and a lovely smile, complains that everyone cheats on the site. She gets the impression that the men copy and paste each other's profiles, so they all sound the same. "The men are non-smokers or rarely smoke, do sports three times a week, all have master's degrees, only drink two glasses of fine Bordeaux, love travelling around Italy and Asia, upload photos taken when they were ten years younger, and say they're still looking for the love of their life. And they all want a beautiful, intelligent woman."

Jaimelavie ("Ilovelife"), 65, agrees: "The profiles are all idealized and therefore fake." The reality is quite different. When she began to exchange messages, the comments she received were often aggressive. One of the men she contacted for a chat asked her how she had the nerve to join a dating site "with a face like that!" She was traumatized and swapped her profile picture for another shot taken ten years earlier. I point out that this is asking for trouble. No, she replies. When one man invited her for coffee, she was the one who got a nasty surprise. He'd also used a shot taken ten years ago, in Egypt—he looked handsome, strong, and tanned, which impressed her. But the man who sat down opposite her had lost ten kilos and seemed old. He was wearing a threadbare jacket and looked terrible. She paid for her coffee and left. The next man she met was from a town in northern France and was looking for an intelligent woman with a good retirement plan. His motivation was clear, at least. She suggested a night at the opera. He booked a hotel room, and they spent the weekend together, but nothing happened. He attempted to kiss her, but she felt completely cold towards him. "You have to understand," she tells me, "I haven't slept with anyone for seven years!"

Josie, 70, adds that "all the guys only have one thing on their minds—sex." She tried to make contact with men her own age, but they all replied that they were looking for a younger woman. Then one day, Cestbienmoi ("Yesitsme") got in touch with her. He claimed to be 69 but was actually 75. His wife had left him, and he hated being alone. They exchanged messages for a couple of weeks, then talked on the phone. He sounded young and cheerful. That persuaded her to meet him for lunch. He seemed very kind and generous. Above all, he was looking for a companion, someone to "spend evenings with by the fire, talking and cuddling." Josie told herself there was no point in being too fussy. After six months on the site, she was losing heart. She still sees Cestbienmoi from time to time, and they are developing a lovely friendship, which she likes.

Angelina, 64, a beautiful, bubbly brunette, admits she claims to be 58 on the site. She's already changed her profile twice, because despite her lovely photo she wasn't getting much traffic. A girlfriend convinced her to lie about her age, since she looks younger anyway. The effect was instantaneous, and she received dozens of messages. One of them really caught her eye because he practiced yoga. She'd said she wanted to meet someone "with a spiritual side." They fell for each other immediately. She tells us she wanted to come to this evening to "encourage the girls." It is possible to find a good match.

Églantine, 70, explains she's decided to leave the site. She's spent two years on it trying to find her soulmate, and the experience has helped her "say goodbye to the idea of meeting someone." She says it has made her see things more clearly, and she is wiser for it. In the end, she doesn't think being single is too bad. And she concludes by saying, "If luck knocks on my door, I'll open it!"

A constant stream of lovers

FLORENCE, 69, TALKS about her experience. Twice divorced, she's been living alone for five years. Since she retired, her life has never been so busy, and she's kept herself occupied with her children, grandchildren, volunteer work, and women's club. She's had a few flings and made a few good friends, but so far the soulmate she's been hoping to meet has eluded her. She's grown used to being alone and is not looking for a man to live with day in, day out, but a good companion: a kind-hearted man who will whisk her off for the weekend and take her on holiday. A loving friendship, perhaps. But she hasn't found him yet and is wondering why. Is she too busy, too demanding? Are her expectations too high? A psychoanalyst friend once told her that women like her, who admire their fathers too much, can never find a man who is good enough.

Another friend persuaded her to join a dating site. She resisted for a long time, saying she'd rather leave it to chance, then decided to do it, *just to see*. Her friend pointed out that nowadays chance manifests itself on dating sites!

So she set about writing up her profile with a wry smile. It's a difficult exercise, as it forces you to introduce yourself and say what you're looking for. It's also quite brutal, because in a certain sense it reduces you to an object of desire that men will look at the way they look at products on a supermarket shelf. Women do the same, of course. Florence wrote a detailed profile that was more or less honest, accompanied by some attractive recent photos showing her beautiful smile and lovely wrinkles. She also chose a photo of herself lying on a sun lounger in a swimsuit, just to show that her body wasn't bad either. The first man to contact her left a message saying "You're the sexiest sexagenarian on AW."

"He probably has no idea how good that made me feel," she says.

In response to the question "What are you expecting from AW?" she replied, "I'm looking for the three As: Attraction, Affection, Admiration." She went on to say that she didn't like men who were tight-fisted or pessimistic, and that she liked making love.

Every evening, Florence and her friend would read their messages and visit the profiles of men whose photos they liked. They laughed as they scrolled through the shots, judging, criticizing, and commenting on them. "This one has a gorgeous face! That one looks sad, ugly, too old … look at what he's wearing! And the way he's posing in front of a sailboat, or by Inle Lake, or in a ski outfit, or on a golf course!" A few days later they decided to reply to one or two messages. Florence picked a man with a good-looking, rugged, bronzed face, who was the same age as she was. There was something sensual about him that she found attractive. She sent him a message telling him so, and he answered immediately. He suggested they go out for coffee at Les Éditeurs, a café-restaurant in Paris near the Odéon national theater. He added that he'd never met a woman on the site who'd been brave enough to say she liked sex in such a direct way. This intrigued him. And he also wanted to get to know her.

He was in fact a handsome man, and their mutual attraction was obvious. They kissed on the second date. Florence invited him to her house in Normandy, and they made love all night long. She nicknamed him her "master of love" because he understood women and knew how to give them pleasure. She felt ten years younger. They took a trip to Venice, went skiing in the Alps, and had a romantic getaway in La Rochelle. In the bedroom things were going really well, but elsewhere they started to get complicated. He came from a very different world, was penniless, and calculated the cost of everything, which she couldn't bear. He spent hours watching TV, which she hated. He was often miserable and had no sense of humor. In short, after two months, she came to her senses. They were completely wrong for each other, and she realized that belonging to the same social class and sharing the same tastes were important after all. She wondered how she could have thrown herself headlong into such a silly affair. She needed to "feel like a woman again," and the best thing about this man was that he was a very good lover. They continued to have sex for two more months, until he left her abruptly—probably because, since he was more experienced than she was, he'd realized their relationship was going nowhere. She thought the way he left her was extremely rude and rather caddish, especially since he took off with a bottle of champagne.

Did the experience put Florence off her quest for true love? Not at all—she got straight back in the saddle, returned to the dating site, and met one man after another.

Letendre ("Mr Gentle") lived up to his username. She loved the way he kissed her constantly and talked to her about the contemporary works of art he exhibited in his gallery. But although he was five years younger than her, he behaved like an old bachelor, which she found annoying. And he pointed out that it was dangerous to say in her profile that she liked making love! She'd be better off letting her lovers find out for themselves. So she changed her profile.

Next she fell for Alsacien, the former boss of a major food corporation, because he was confident and self-possessed, qualities she liked in a man. They spent a weekend in Istanbul, but he didn't lay a finger on her, much to her surprise—despite sleeping in the same bed! He said he needed time before he could touch her. She might have given him the time, had he been nicer. But he turned out to be mean, negative about everything, and "constantly complaining." She couldn't stand it, and they left it at that.

Then there was Titan, a small man who certainly didn't live up to his username. He was slightly older than Florence and wasn't good-looking, but she immediately liked the way he touched her. He was a gentle man. She loved cuddling up to him. Their affair didn't last either, because he wanted to move to south-west France, and she quickly found out he wasn't completely over his ex.

To sum up, Florence has had a constant stream of lovers. She could carry on that way, too, because she's a very beautiful woman, sensual and feminine, and men obviously find her attractive. But this hopeless search for the perfect man has exhausted her. "No, clearly you can't meet your soulmate in this kind of environment where love is commodified. I've learned a lot about myself and my body, about the sexual and emotional misery and complexity of single men and women of my age on their senseless quest for love. I'm still convinced that the best way to meet someone is by chance, when you're ready for it. I've realized that, rather than focusing on finding a companion that life may or may not bring you, it's more important to improve your ability to be intimate with the people you love and who matter."

In the end she decided to go back to an old lover, who unfortunately was married, but who makes her feel good and sees to it that he meets with her every now and then. She tells herself that on balance, it's better to be single than in a bad relationship.

The temptation of polyamory

MARCELA, 67, SHARES the story of the relationship she had with a man ten years her junior—a relationship she felt was very immature.

I've nicknamed her Marcela because she reached a turning point in her love affair with Christian after reading an interview with Marcela Iacub in the French daily newspaper *Libération*.[21] Divorced for seven years, she is the mother of two and a grandmother, journalist, and feminist with an interest in sustainable development and the global-justice movement. She lives alone and has had a few casual lovers, but her sex life was in the doldrums until she fell violently in love with a man in his 50s who she met in Lyon at the annual forum hosted by the organization *Dialogues en humanité*.

There was instant chemistry between them, she says, "from the moment we first saw each other." He was a handsome, sensual man with kind eyes. During the breaks they talked non-stop about the topic that had brought them to Lyon. They swapped email addresses and phone numbers, and she returned home feeling quite flustered by the encounter. She wrote to tell him as soon as she got back to Paris. She wanted to see him again. He felt the same way. They agreed to meet for lunch the following week and declared their mutual attraction. But it was summer time, and they both had holiday plans. At this point Marcela gave herself a reality check. Christian was married and obviously attached to his family. But neither of them had any moral objections in principle. They decided to wait till the end of the summer and to write to each other in the meantime.

While Christian was on holiday with his wife and children in Brittany, he sent her a long email in which he wrote, "Life's too short to miss out on the things that make this journey so rich and exhilarating." He felt he had something "fundamental" to share with her. What form would this take? He didn't know, but hoped they could "make it up together." She replied that she was ready but asked him how he saw things. Then he sent her a text about erotic friendship. He was frank with her: he felt attracted to her, and being unable to "fully commit to love," since he had a wife and teenage children who still needed him, he suggested they have a gentle, affectionate relationship that could even be erotic, but not exclusive. Marcela replied saying she was afraid she was too sensual and physical to stay within the limits of a lighthearted loving friendship. She knew herself too well. If there was intimacy, she would become deeply attached and surrender to it. Then she told him there was still time to stop, if he was scared of going too far. But she was prepared to take a gamble on this unexpected relationship, which had come out of nowhere.

Did this expression of desire in her response fire him up? Because the tone of the messages he sent her afterwards, in the middle of the night, around three or four o'clock in the morning, when he was probably suffering from insomnia, changed. They were blatantly erotic messages, whispers of love in the night. He wrote that he was magnetically drawn to her, that he wanted to kiss and caress her, feel her skin, make her quiver. Then he sent her poems and messages expressing his unbridled love for her. Marcela recalls that when she received them, she told herself that this man couldn't be making love with his wife anymore. She felt confused and excited, but a voice inside her told her not to get carried away. The best thing now would be to do the deed.

"I'm waiting for you, I want you," she wrote. A window in the middle of the summer enabled them to meet at long last, and their virtual relationship became physical and sexual. The three days they spent making love were exquisite. She wasn't disappointed. Christian told her he had been initiated into Tantra, and he was clearly very experienced in erotic techniques. They discovered their pleasure gently and slowly, just as she liked it. It's worth pointing out that she had hardly had sex in five years. She trusted him and surrendered, sensing he was really in love. She still has fond memories of this romantic getaway.

After they returned home, however, he sent her a distraught message. He said he felt completely lost, torn apart. He was in love with Marcela but attached to his wife and not ready to leave her. He was wondering how he could make room for their affair. He was suddenly afraid of hurting his wife. "He'd been turning the dilemma over and over in his mind, trying to see if there was a way he could stay with his wife without giving up his love affair with me. He felt strongly that the fact that he loved me didn't mean he no longer loved his wife." When Marcela received the letter, she was in the middle of reading the *Libération* article entitled "Why not have several erotic friendships at the same time?" It argued the case for multiple relationships, "relationships that could last a lifetime alongside your main one." Iacub even put forward the idea that it was the only way couples could stay together. So Marcela suggested to Christian that they embark on a polyamorous relationship.[22] After all, hadn't he hinted that he subscribed to this kind of lifestyle? They'd had long discussions about open, non-exclusive relationships that were transparent and responsible. It wasn't "her or me, but her and me"—a sort of loving inclusivity that implied being honest about the existence of the person outside the central relationship.

"I told him I was a free-spirited kind of woman and not the sort who would suffocate a man by constantly demanding his presence. I didn't need to be with him all the time. I was willing to share him. But I wanted to exist and be seen by his side. I wanted our relationship to be socially acknowledged. You know," she adds, looking me straight in the eye, "I've already been involved in a secret affair, where I was the mistress on the side. I know myself too well, and it's not for me. I don't like the idea of the man in my life having to lie and tell stories. I think I'm worth more than that."

Marcela told him she would respect his lifestyle, understand that others needed him and his love, and work around his limited time, provided she felt other people also saw *her* as his partner. Since he was a progressive, unconventional man, she didn't see why he wouldn't openly take on two relationships that were equally important. Christian listened but said nothing.

"We spent a second romantic weekend together, which was lighthearted and sensual. He joined me on holiday, and I introduced him to some of my friends. It was another step forward in our relationship. He seemed relaxed, and I thought my friends liked him." Most importantly, their second encounter confirmed the sensual connection they'd created between them. "It was so unusual that the next week I felt like singing out loud in gratitude the whole time. I don't think I'd ever been so happy." So it was like a dagger to her heart when she received another email from Christian saying he felt "torn apart inside" and clearly stating that he didn't want to risk hurting his wife by telling her about their relationship. He suggested they have a secret erotic friendship like all the others he'd had until then. Marcela took it very badly. She thought it smacked of cowardice and that he was running away from the situation. "How could he send me those passionate messages in the middle of the night while his wife was sleeping in the bed just a few meters away? How could he declare his love for me, only to backtrack so quickly?"

Marcela still seems very hurt as she tells me all this. She seems to feel betrayed somehow by a man who had presented himself as a modern, open-minded person who subscribed to the polyamorous lifestyle but who ultimately behaved like a guilty child who couldn't take responsibility for his actions. "In his last email, Christian told me he had started seeing a therapist again and apologized for leading me to believe we could have a love affair he was unable to conduct," says Marcela, who still sounds devastated.

Was she right to have been so demanding? As I listen to her, it strikes me that conducting an erotic friendship outside a committed relationship isn't that simple and that to be happy within a polyamorous lifestyle, you need to work on yourself in a way few couples do. You have to face feelings of jealousy, your desire to possess others, your fear of hurting them, your guilt. It's pretty rare to be able to do that.

"To be happy within a polyamorous lifestyle, you need to work on yourself in a way few couples do."

But maybe some older people are able to do this because they have grown wiser over the years. I'm thinking of those men and women who instinctively know their partner has a special, even intimate, relationship with someone else and choose to look the other way, as long as that relationship doesn't affect their own.

Meeting Marcela made me want to immerse myself in the books of Françoise Simpère.[23] I was intrigued by the

Canadian writer's open challenge to monogamy. In a recent interview, she calmly argues that there is more than one type of relationship and that monogamous couples are not necessarily happy.[24] "One couple in three will separate or divorce, and those who stay together are often bored with each other." Why not have a strong family unit (if you have children) and multiple partners? Simpère thinks it's possible and has experienced it herself. "We're always being told that biodiversity is essential to nature and the environment, and flexibility is key in the workplace, yet in love we're supposed to practice 'monoculture,' which drains and depletes feelings just as it does soil!" Of course, reading this we know full well that the '"biodiversity in love" Simpère is referring to has been secretly practiced by couples since time began, and infidelity has always existed.

What sets apart polyamory from infidelity, which is based on lies and hypocrisy, or even from swinging and open relationships, is that the relationships are transparent but not flaunted. Both people know that their partner has other lovers or other erotic friendships, but they respect these extramarital relationships and don't try to intrude. Each one has their own secret garden. "It seems perfectly natural for the man I love (and with whom I may have children) to be happy with me as well as with others. In my view, love is not about possession, but about caring for each other and wanting each other to be happy above all else. I'm not asking for an exclusive relationship." What characterizes this open-minded attitude to love and friendship is an honesty about the existence of these relationships, as well as a total respect for the quality of intimacy and the way it is experienced. Françoise

Simpère herself says she has been involved in a loving friendship with a man she has made love to only five times in 25 years. The most important thing is that she feels free to behave in a way that's right for the relationship, without feeling guilty.

• • •

CHAPTER THREE

Couples who stand the test of time

What makes a couple? What enables people to stay together? How do you recapture that "first-time feeling"?

• • •

M OVING ON FROM older adults living through a "second adolescence," I'm now going to investigate couples of "mature" 60-somethings who have stood the test of time, those who have managed to live through crises and have stayed together. Often, the price they pay for the longevity of their relationship is the end of their sex life. As long as they mutually agree to move on to "something different," all is well. If you're happy no longer making love, that's fine. In the following pages, I'll be looking at what keeps couples happy over time, whether or not they still make love. Also, what makes a couple a couple? What binds a couple together?

Deciding to be happy

SOCIETY HAS A rather rigid and simplistic view of ageing couples. People think they find each other hard to bear and get bored in each other's company, and that nothing goes on between them anymore. They're wrong. Whether they've been a couple for a long time or are on their second go, when they reach their 70s, experience makes them more attentive and less demanding. They have learned from the past.

One of my friends told me a secret recently: "I've simply decided to be happy." Life isn't always perfect with his wife, and there are areas in which he's not completely in tune with her, but as desire and love still exist in their relationship, he reckons that his decision to be happy provides a good basis for their relationship to grow deeper in an atmosphere of trust. And my own observations prove him right. The act of showing your partner you're happy with them—because you have decided to be—instils trust in the relationship.

People will argue that you can't just decide to be happy. I disagree. French philosopher Émile-Auguste Chartier, commonly known as Alain, said: "Be happy: that is true happiness." We can decide to see life in its most favorable light rather than pick out everything that's wrong with it. We can decide to focus on what we like in our partner rather than expecting them to live up to our ideal. It's a personal decision that anyone can make at any age. In the "growing old happily" seminars I regularly run, I ask the question: can we decide to grow old happily? The answer is yes. People aged 80 to 100 tell me that it's a decision they make every morning when they wake up. What will I focus on today? My aches and pains? My sadness that my children don't call me often enough? Or the joy I feel when I go for a walk in the park or countryside, when someone smiles at me, when a neighbor makes a friendly gesture, or when I listen to a Bach cantata?

For couples fortunate enough to still be together, this vow to be happy is the key to a certain happy glow that is not as rare as we might think. But how do you reconcile that vow with the vow to maintain desire? What place does sexual intimacy have in the relationship? A couple, whether married or not, is defined by the social presupposition of a shared sex life. But we know that for the majority of people, the older they get, the less true that is.

"The act of showing your partner you're happy with them—because you have decided to be—instils trust in the relationship."

When I meet the author Éric-Emmanuel Schmitt at the Mantua Literary Festival, we speak about waning desire between partners.[25] "Desire is autonomous," he tells me. "It just happens to you. The same as fate." So we aren't free to desire at all. The only freedom we have is accepting or not to love the man or woman we desire. Éric adds that love has nothing to do with desire—they are two separate things. We know for a fact that couples can carry on loving each other without necessarily desiring each other anymore.

"But isn't there a way of maintaining desire in a relationship?" I ask him. "It's extremely difficult," Éric replies, "because the need for security and the wish to make the relationship last cause desire to fade, even to disappear. We need a strategy to deal with insecurity," he concludes, "because closeness, though reassuring, weakens desire. We need to recreate that 'first-time feeling.'"

That "first-time feeling"—what a lovely expression! I read about it in Esther Perel's book on erotic intelligence.[26] She advises cultivating distance in the relationship, bringing an element of risk back into the security, reinjecting mystery into the familiar, and recreating the spice, playfulness, and romance that first connected the couple.

"Love has nothing to do with desire—they
are two separate things."

We will never know our loved ones inside out. Desire is proportionate to the degree of mystery our partner still has in our eyes. An 80-year-old romantic I know tells me he is still learning new things about his wife, even after 50 years of living together. He comes across as so young when we talk! He tells me that for ten years he has been "cultivating the spirit of childhood"—that is, looking differently at life and at his partner. This involves exploring the intimate. The intimate, in the sense that François Jullien describes it: "far from noisy love."[27] In other words, the ability to share with your partner your innermost being, what happens and unfolds deep within yourself, as well as an interest in their intimate being. This has nothing to do with intrusion—rather, it is a permanent curiosity about the other, a predisposition to appreciate what is deeply mysterious and unexpected about them. This attitude keeps desire alive and frustration and weariness at bay. "Every day, there's something new," says the 80-year-old romantic.

Being able to daydream side by side

WHAT KEEPS COUPLES together over time? That is the question that Claude Habib asks in a book I greatly enjoyed: *Le goût de la vie commune* ("Opting for Coupledom").[28] It is a lovely argument in favor of coupledom. Being a "matrimonialist," she says, doesn't mean "approving of confinement." We can be in a relationship and feel free. Not free to look *elsewhere*, in the sense of having a lover or a mistress, but free inside ourselves. One aspect of that freedom is being able to *escape through our thoughts*. To experience that as a couple, you have to be able to be bored together. I like how she praises boredom: "Boredom isn't an obstacle to coupledom [...] it forms the basis of conjugal life, its *sine qua non*."[29] It is "the basis of peace, like the soft silt at the bottom of the lake in which we immerse ourselves to recharge our batteries. Through that invisible exercise, that inner swimming, we achieve self-control [...] and are able to make progress within ourselves. Not progress like we do in a career, nor progress along a path mapped out by others, but progress in an unpredictable way—like a shoal of fish in the sea—which presupposes the existence of an inner world."[30]

"You have to be able to be bored together."

An "inner world"! That's what this is all about. Older couples who are still happy together are the couples who are willing to get bored together because they have an inner life. Few people talk about how precious boredom is, Habib says, because it's embarrassing: "Nothing is more common or more widespread. It's the grayness of life, the opposite of sparkle. How do you get rid of it?" We obviously have to differentiate between tedium brought on by confinement, which is toxic, and idle time, when you can get in touch with yourself. The latter is the key to happiness in a couple. You can spend all day with each other, without talking, without doing anything in particular, in a kind of shared emptiness. Each person is wrapped up in their own thoughts, but the thoughts communicate in the ether, you could say. Being able to do that in a relationship is a sign of love. And of trust.

I've just spoken to one of my musician friends on the phone. He told me he has always loved sex and that eroticism is still very much alive in him. But not in his wife. She has moved on and doesn't like making love anymore. So they no longer desire each other. Their married life carries on as if nothing has changed. They share everyday things and respect each other's interests—music for him, literature for her—but they no longer have physical contact. They sleep together but don't touch each other. Is he okay with that? No, of course not. The lover in him, secretly nostalgic for sexual pleasure, is suffering. On several occasions he has had the urge to approach a woman he was attracted to. He felt his body stir and yearned to take her in his arms, surrender to lust, and experience the deep joy of sexual union. The lover in him is indeed very much alive.

But he has weighed up the risk of having an extramarital affair and doesn't feel capable of having a secret relationship, as so many men do. He loves his wife and doesn't want to risk hurting her. So he has found a way to satisfy the lover in him. He has erotic dreams and wakes up from them feeling incredibly alive. They are about a woman whose appearance, face, and body often change but who always gives herself to him in the same way. He calls her his "anima." They take each other passionately, and when he wakes up, he is always surprised to find he has had a wet dream, like a teenager. He has started talking to his erotic anima. He sends her poems and writes her letters. Thanks to the power of his active imagination and of connecting with his dreams in writing, he is thrilled to find that the woman answers him back. He could be taken for a madman. But he isn't. Through reading Jung, he has learned that men and women can connect with their inner personalities. His own inner erotic life has the same power and reality as the one he could lead externally.

Cultivating harmony for harmony's sake

IS A COUPLE a couple because they live together? "That isn't a prerequisite," Claude Habib replies. "There are couples who live together, but there's a gulf between them. There are also couples, dubbed Living Apart Together (LAT) by American sociologists, who share great intimacy but have chosen not to live together. Their living space isn't a geographical place, it's *inside* them. What makes a couple a couple is the decision to put your partner at the center of your life."

According to Habib, what keeps couples together over time is the "desire to cultivate harmony for harmony's sake." Staying in sync with each other, in other words.

Moving through time like dancers moving on a dance floor. I can't help thinking of the pleasure I experience watching old couples who know each other inside out dance together, their graceful steps completely in sync and inner happiness written all over their serious, thoughtful faces. We can't help being deeply moved by this togetherness, when the anticipation of one partner meets the leadership of the other. This synchronization involves the body, eyes, and rhythm, giving rise to a very erotic kind of desire.

"What makes a couple a couple is the decision to put your partner at the center of your life."

Another kind of synchrony—telepathy, thinking the same thing at the same time—produces similar results and still involves Eros, sexual pleasure. It's that feeling of surprise when you realize you've guessed what the other was thinking, when you kiss them tenderly on their neck or snuggle up to them, just as they are secretly wanting it. Isn't that surprise, the result of silent connectedness, a form of orgasm? The realization that you are on the same wavelength, invisible but no less real, produces incredible pleasure. This kind of complicity is a far cry from that jaded feeling you get when you think you know everything there is to know about your partner and your life together. This unpredictability, the surprise you experience when your bodies and minds unite, is the source of sensual pleasure.

It is often when a relationship breaks down or when one partner dies that we realize what made the couple last.

We sorely miss the wonderful connectedness that came from giving ourselves to the other person and from receiving their attention. We realize we soon get bored with our own company when we live alone. Afterwards, we appreciate all the things that made our life together so lovely, like the way we used to look forward to our partner coming home: "He'll be back soon and we'll have a cup of tea. Can't wait for this evening and for him to cook for me. We could go for a walk in the garden. I can hear the key in the lock." The mere possibility of the other's presence, of their return, gives us a little boost as we process how we're feeling.[31] Ultimately, this *subtle expansion*, which is rooted in trust and reciprocity, is what gives life as a couple its value. "Even if you're far away, I imagine you're thinking of me just as I'm thinking of you."

But can this connectedness be experienced outside an exclusive, faithful relationship? I'm thinking of the "secret" a couple shared with me recently. He's 75 and she's 72. Whenever they need to talk about what's wrong in their relationship, they make an appointment with each other. They sit down opposite each other, hold hands, and look into each other's eyes. It is a posture of giving and receiving. They offer themselves to each other. The position alone shows that neither party is judging. Whoever has something to say talks, knowing they won't be interrupted. Their partner listens to them. And each of them will mull over what the other has said in the hours and days to come. This very intimate ritual has its rules. The person who is listening acknowledges what the other says without replying, justifying themselves, or judging. If they really need to talk, they ask their partner's permission to do so. This approach creates respect. It isn't a discussion or a settling of scores.

The ritual does them a lot of good. It doesn't give rise to arguments, grievances, or misunderstandings. It gives rise to a unique form of tenderness because they feel they are being heard by their partner. They are a true couple.

• • •

CHAPTER FOUR

Couples who have had enough of sex

Why do some older people stop having sex? Can desire be revived?

● ● ●

SEVENTY PERCENT OF French people aged over 65 have apparently decided to stop devoting energy to sex. Sex belonged to their youth and middle years. These couples fall into two groups: those who have grown tired of sex over time, and those whose sexual appetite has simply been satisfied once and for all.

It's easy to spot those who are tired of sex. They were never that into it. They give the excuse that they don't feel attractive enough anymore—as if that's a natural consequence of their changing bodies—to focus their attention elsewhere. This gradual abandonment seems to take place naturally. The main point is that neither party feels frustrated or lost. They get used to having separate bedrooms or sleeping side by side without touching, like brother and sister. This change in their situation means at least two things: the couple's sex life was never important, and they stopped making love well before they turned 60. The man sometimes used to play the field, most often in secret, to satisfy his sexual needs. The woman adapts fairly easily to their new set-up by concentrating instead on her friendships, family, children, and grandchildren.

Then there are those who have had their fill of making love. They've had lots of sex and just don't feel like it anymore. But their fondness for skin-to-skin contact never really goes away. I have lots of friends in their 70s who are in relationships, and even though they no longer have sex like they used to when they were young, they sleep naked next to each other and still like that physical connection. Love flows between them.

We've decided not to have sex anymore

JEAN-LOUIS HAS JUST turned 65. We've known each other for a long time through our work with people with HIV, as we founded a non-profit together to help them.[32] Our work has created a strong bond that has withstood time, even if we hardly see each other now. When I met him 30 years ago, he was a director, an actor, and a homosexual. He had stirred up his share of passions, was extraordinarily dynamic and generous. He is still one of the most creative and vibrant people I know.

Jean-Louis was stunning, with the body of a faun and a rare magnetism. His commitment to HIV-positive people began with his unwavering support of his boyfriend at the time, Serge, whom he loved and cared for until the day he died. I admired him greatly, and I remember how attentive he was, getting up every night to bathe, massage, and soothe his sick partner. Then one day he met a woman who did the same volunteer work as him and fell in love. He changed careers and became a psychotherapist, training medical staff to deal with patients in a humane and tactful manner. He married Michelle, and they had three daughters. I remember him saying that, with her, he had finally found what he had been looking for for a long time. He had never been happier. His is certainly an unconventional life.[33] I don't know any other man who switched from homosexuality to heterosexuality like that in his prime of life.

But what is even more unusual, I think, is that when he reached early old age (in other words, his 60th birthday), he and his wife decided to stop having sex. I was so surprised that I asked if he would agree to be interviewed for this book. I am still deeply moved by the trust he put in me by saying yes.

"We haven't 'made love' for two years. The desire is still there, but it has taken a different form. Our lovemaking has taken a back seat. It isn't as important as our moments of infinite tenderness, our general conversation, our day-to-day lives, our children's education, our work, and our discussions about current affairs."

Jean-Louis: "The desire is still there, but it has taken a different form."

Jean-Louis says that Michelle and he don't feel any frustration. Their sexuality has changed. Things were crazy when they first met. They had "that constant need to be together, to make love like wild animals, which calmed down over time." Their sexuality has gone through many stages, but none really instigated by them. "They've happened naturally," he explains. Their current situation—no longer making love—is just one of those stages. And they're happy with it. They have balance in their life. "Our love for each other is still changing, being fine-tuned. It surprises us by taking on new colors as time passes and binding us together more strongly than ever."

Jean-Louis tells me that at the age of 65 he "still looks at women's physiques." Sometimes they have an effect on him—their aura, the way they are, or how they do things. "They arouse feelings of tenderness, protectiveness, or love in me, but not lust." It's as if his sexual energy, which used to be so strong, is now shared across the rest of his life and his activities and on the attention he focuses on his family, friends, and other people.

As I listen to him, I sense something very different from the sad abandonment of sex I've come across in other people. "I haven't abandoned sex," he says. "It's because I've had my fill, because I used to live my sex life in the fast lane, that I can move on to something else. I'm no longer obsessed with sex like I was when I was younger. My desires have changed over time. The way I look at people is no longer marred by interpretation, expectation, or desire. My intentions are clearer. I don't have ulterior motives. I feel more available for the people around me."

What Jean-Louis describes is essentially a wonderful example of sublimation. Which is why there's no frustration. More importantly, everything remains open, and anything is possible in this unique love story.

"We've felt free since the day we met. Anything is still possible. It could all begin again. Nothing's dead. This freedom enables us to constantly share our deepest feelings and to trust each other. I've never had this level of trust with anyone else. I can tell Michelle anything because she knows how to listen. Better than listen—what I tell her resonates with her."

Michelle sums up this freedom in a lovely way: "We touch each other tenderly, stroke each other, listen to each other, whisper to each other, discuss things, brush against each other, talk things over, look for each other, find each other, meet each other, share, soothe each other, give things a go, give everything a go, love each other!"

It takes me a while to assimilate what they're telling me. It seems like such an unusual thing for a couple in their prime to say. "But if you still have that physical contact and you sleep in the same bed, don't you ever feel the need to be united more closely? Physically, sexually?" I ask, afraid of being too intrusive.

Jean-Louis calmly replies that the very idea of making love exhausts him. He says all his sexual experiences have satisfied his hunger. His sexuality is still alive, but he doesn't miss it at all. "We sleep together, and when we snuggle up we're happy because holding each other doesn't require anything more than that. Having said that, there's nothing to stop us from going further, and sometimes we do have a more sexual, passionate embrace. But it's always full of tenderness. We love our new kind of intimate connection that involves different feelings and ways of touching."

Fading desire

AS ÉRIC-EMMANUEL SCHMITT pointed out, "You can't choose when you feel desire." It just happens to you.

I came across an article in *Libération* featuring the conversation of a fictitious couple whose desire for each other has faded.[34] According to the author, it's one of the most taboo subjects in a relationship. Admitting to, facing, and talking about a loss of sexual desire is very difficult. He shares a dialogue that few couples dare to have, in bed one night:

A: This is awful.
B: It will come back.
A: No, it won't, we haven't had sex for six months.
B: It will come back. We're tired. We've got issues.

The dialogue continues. The man reminds the woman that when they used to have sex, they had even bigger worries than now—no job, a dying mother. Then he asks the right question: "Don't you think we're tired because we aren't excited? When we wanted sex all the time, we were never tired." There it is: they don't want it anymore. Then we read that, according to a survey, tiredness is the number-one reason people don't make love anymore. The second reason, that the children might hear, obviously doesn't concern sexagenarians anymore, unless perhaps they are on holiday in the same house as their children.

Not only do they no longer want to have sex, but this couple has a very pessimistic take on life: "We're old. We eat, we watch a film, we feel like dying, we don't have sex anymore, and we always sleep badly. And so it goes on, from bad to worse, until we die."

They wonder what solutions there are to their fading desire. Getting drunk? Taking Viagra? Sex toys? Sleeping

with someone else to check if the machinery's still working properly? Surprising your partner, wearing exciting
underwear, giving gifts, being thoughtful? Not discussing the awful day you've had in bed at night? Behavioral
therapy? Going to a swingers' party? Fantasizing about
someone else? Taking a lover, but not telling your partner?
They think of every conceivable solution.

Then at last they ask the right question: What is desire?
Have sexual liberation and internet porn damaged it? "Sex
has become a series of sexual acts to try out ... If doing 'it'
like that is continuing to make love, anyone can do it. You
can vary things with as many scenarios and gadgets as you
want, it's still sexual intercourse."

Would the couple actually like the opposite: to desire
each other like when they first met? Desire conflicts with
the obligation to climax. It conflicts with sex as something
to consume. The more we want to revive desire, the more it
disappears. Desire cannot be controlled.

The conversation ends on a delightful note: "We can't
force 'it' to come back, but that doesn't mean 'it'—desire—
which is completely free, won't come back!"

Resisting the obligation to climax

DESIRE CONFLICTS WITH the obligation to climax. One
way it might conflict is by going on strike.

Just as I was getting up to say goodbye to François Parpaix after a whole afternoon discussing sexuality in the
over-60s and how to regain intimacy, he started giving me his thoughts on today's 20-somethings who have
lost their libido and what kind of older generation they

would make. He isn't optimistic; he has observed that young people are showing a decline in their ability to have erotic relationships.

"What does intimacy mean for these young people who flaunt their private lives on Facebook, who don't have any real friends, and who become aggressive if they don't get everything they want straightaway? Who get drunk, smoke joints, seek solitary excitement, and spend their evenings alone on the internet, including on porn sites? Who withdraw into their shells, sulk, and isolate themselves? Their parents are anti-models. These young people haven't seen their parents kiss, gaze lovingly at each other, or demonstrate intimacy for ages."

"Desire conflicts with the obligation to climax."

François told me that 20- to 25-year-olds go and see him because they have zero libido, and sex with their girlfriends isn't working. But he also added, "The ones coming to see me are the crème de la crème, because by coming to see me they are taking responsibility for themselves." What kind of over-60s will they make? Won't they show sexual and emotional immaturity? Tragic loneliness?

Then he told me about an article he had just read about millions of young Japanese people who are losing interest in sex and love.[35] It's a new phenomenon, and one that might travel. *Sekkusu shinai shokogun* ("celibacy syndrome") is seen by the Japanese government as a looming national catastrophe. According to a survey taken in 2013 by the Japan Family Planning Association, 45 percent of Japanese women aged 16 to 24 "are not interested in or despise sexual contact." They are becoming independent and ambitious, and sexual relationships are clearly perceived as an obstacle to their career plans. Marriage is "the grave of their hard-won careers." Romantic commitment "seems to represent burden and drudgery."[36]

Mendokusai, they say. Which means "too troublesome" or "I can't be bothered." Their phobia of romantic relationships is shared by Japanese men. An increasing number of them still live with their parents and have replaced sexual intercourse with virtual relationships and watching online porn.[37] Men there are often heard saying they prefer virtual girlfriends to real ones.

Some Japanese people do get married and have a child, but once the baby comes along, 40 percent of couples say they stop having sex. Increasingly they turn towards egocentric eroticism. Shared sexuality has ceased being a factor in self-fulfilment and relationship success. The auto-eroticism market has truly taken off.

Demographers estimate that Japan will have lost a third of its population by 2060 and that slowly but surely the country is evolving into a type of society that has only been depicted in science fiction. Will this phenomenon spread to the rest of the world? Are we witnessing the birth of a new form of self-centered, auto-erotic humanity, in which sex—the symbol of relationships—will eventually disappear?

According to a recent article in *L'Express*, more and more young people are showing a lack of interest in sex and physical love.[38] They simply don't feel desire anymore. There is even an international Asexual Awareness Week and an association for asexuals, the Asexuality Visibility and Education Network (AVEN). Unlike abstinence, asexuality is not a choice. It is the state of not experiencing sexual attraction. On forums for asexuals, they give themselves the nickname "ace" and resent being labeled sick, frustrated, or waiting for the right person. For them, their lack of sexual desire isn't a problem. They don't feel fear or disgust, just indifference. Ace activists refer to their absence of sexual desire as a "sexual orientation" and explain that it's fully compatible with having feelings of love.

Asexuality has probably always existed but just wasn't given a name before. Some of the spinsters and bachelors of yesteryear may well have been asexual. They lived marginal lives and grew old alone. What could be the psychological cause of this lack of interest in sex? An unresolved Oedipus complex? A childhood trauma? What does it mean in a world where sexuality is promoted all over the media? We hear people say, "too much sex kills sex." There may well be some truth to this observation.

. . .

CHAPTER FIVE

Solitude and freedom

How do older women deal with living on their own?
And can they still be sexual under those circumstances?

· · ·

ALONGSIDE THE REAL and fantasy relationships I've just explored lies solitude. Brigitte Lahaie touched on the subject when we met. "You wouldn't believe the number of single women, aged over and even under 60, who complain about not meeting men! It's the fate of women. Men generally don't remain partner-less for very long."

But do they all complain? Many women are still beautiful and often choose to be alone. Take the 60-year-old who came to tell me after one of my talks that she'd left her husband. "We did it amicably," she added, with a degree of panache. She had been keen to get her freedom back.

Women like her aren't after a potential partner. They want to experience the joys of liberty. She made me think of Sylvie Brunel's novel, which I really enjoyed. Inspired by the lyrics of Led Zeppelin's "Stairway to Heaven," it is a vibrant tribute to women's strength and their ability to enjoy freedom.[39] Women are better than men at living on their own, she says. Loneliness doesn't enter into it. They enjoy doing things on their own and for themselves, and not being accountable to anyone. "Lying diagonally across my bed, turning the light on in the middle of the night to read because I feel like it, deciding how I spend my time without needing approval, stopping to take in a beautiful sunset, going to the cinema without having to let anyone know I'll be late. Not having to justify myself anymore!"

The radiant woman who came to see me after my talk was going to take care of herself and make sure she did what she loved doing. I didn't ask her why she couldn't have experienced all that with her husband, because I knew the answer. Like many couples, they'd lived side by side without probing the depths of their intimacy. They'd gradually drifted apart. When a man who has always worked away from home returns, things are often spoiled.

Forced solitude

BUT OTHER WOMEN have been left by their husbands or partners for someone younger, or they've lost the man they lived with following a long, serious illness.

"I don't like being on my own," says Anne, whose husband left her ten years ago. This pretty 68-year-old has adapted to her solitude but doesn't like it. In the beginning she found it very sad having to eat her breakfast on her own, or coming home after a busy day to a dark, empty apartment. Although she's good-looking, desirable, energetic, and interesting, she hasn't met anyone she would like to live with. This often surprises her friends. "You're beautiful, why haven't you met anyone?" Is she too demanding? Is she still attached to her husband?

Like many women in her situation, Anne decided to register on a reputable dating website. But after a year of disappointing dates, she gave up her search for a man and resolved to accept her situation. No more looking or waiting. Instead, she decided to make the most of what life had to offer. But what life was offering was married men. "I hope you realize all the good men are taken!" a friend declared to her recently. "Experience what you can with them and tell yourself that perhaps you've got the best bit. You don't have to put up with arguments over breakfast or the mediocrity and boredom of daily life."

Anne agreed but hasn't given up her dream of meeting a partner she can fall in love with. To make the best of the situation, she has told herself that she's no doubt going through this period of solitude for a reason. It's teaching her to be truly independent. To enjoy dining alone in the bistro opposite where she lives. It's giving her a sexual freedom that many women around her envy.

Then there's Pierrette (68), who was widowed five years ago. A bereavement support group has really helped her since her husband died. She tells me she's been through several stages. She was so attached to her "man" that she truly thought she would never have a love or sex life again, as she would be unable to find anything as good. In the first few months after his death, she admits to idealizing their relationship; she was convinced that if she ever had another husband, he would be "a poor substitute" for her first one.

Her Catholic friends are rather conventional and disapproving when it comes to the subject of sex. They even believe that widows no longer have the right to a sex life. Pierrette might have agreed, had she not decided to meet up with other women in the same situation as her. When she came out of mourning—which doesn't mean that you forget the one you've lost but that you start wanting to live your own life again—she began to feel like meeting other men. But things weren't that simple. First she wondered if she was still desirable. Then she realized, like Anne, that it wasn't easy to find "decent" single men. As I listen to her, I think about the statistics reporting that 37 percent of widowed and divorced women don't have partners, compared with only 16 percent of men. "You see, men prefer being in a bad relationship than being on their own. They aren't as fussy as we women are. Plus they turn to younger women, because they are racked with fear about growing old. That creates an imbalance."

One of Pierrette's girlfriends encouraged her to give up her search for a companion and to concentrate on all the other opportunities for love that life brings: children, grandchildren, friends. She said things like: "Anyway, the men you'd meet would only think about sex!" Hadn't she herself formed a loving, sensual relationship with a female friend that made her very happy? It was as if she was saying that her same-sex friendship liberated her from the need for a man!

But Pierrette isn't attracted to women and still feels the desire to meet a male partner. She knows that finding love means rekindling her sex life, which doesn't happen at the click of a finger. She's hesitant about joining a dating site, even though some of her girlfriends are trying to persuade her to. She knows she won't find the man she's looking for among her circle of friends. She is surrounded by couples and realizes people categorize her as a single woman—that is, a potential threat and sexual predator. Nobody invites her to dinner anymore, "as if the women, sensing I have *desires*, are instinctively defending their territory."

Daring to give yourself pleasure

I MEET A woman called Sonia, who introduces herself as bisexual and is very comfortable with her sexuality. She grew up in Algeria and dates her sensual awakening back to a very special memory that she's keen to share with us. Her nanny used to take her to the hammam—public baths where women massage each other sensuously with perfumed oils. "All these voluptuous North African women would wrap me in their arms, kiss me, caress me, and rub scented oils into my skin." Sonia is certain that the way the hammam women were with their bodies and their very erotic, feminine tenderness played a key role in shaping the lover she became. She even says those women saved her femininity because her cold, undemonstrative mother wouldn't have helped her discover it. Her first lesbian experience was at the age of 17 with a woman twice her age, who she went on to live with for six years. The woman ended their relationship to go and live with Sonia's best friend, who she had fallen in love with.

After their painful separation, Sonia embarked on a career in the theater, and when she was 26 she met a young man who was "very handsome, cheerful, and loved nature." She lived with him for six years, too. Sonia liked the sensual contact with his body but realized she far preferred making love with a woman. The power of her first sexual feeling, that "sharing of a woman's body," had undoubtedly had an everlasting impact on her sexuality. Yet Sonia refuses to be categorized as a lesbian. "I consider myself to be 'multiple.'" After the break-up with her first male lover, who became a good friend, Sonia had one relationship after another—sometimes with women, sometimes with men, sometimes younger, sometimes older. "I've never left anyone. All my lovers leave me for other people. I've always accepted that they leave me because I love them. I think the people we meet and fall in love with throughout our lives enrich us as human beings."

She has successfully navigated through periods of aloneness. "I remember going to Bali on my own. I saw 70-year-old women working in the fields, and I thought: *How lucky am I to be able to go out and have a coffee on a café terrace, not to be raped, to be free, to be able to marvel at so many things.* It made me realize how fortunate I am." Then, when Sonia was 46, she was diagnosed with cancer. Her energy, optimism, and *joie de vivre* gave her the strength to fight for her life. She'd met a woman 17 years her junior, who supported her during the two years of her illness. She left her as soon as Sonia was declared in remission but has remained a close friend.

As I listen to Sonia telling her story, I'm struck by her resilience: so many break-ups, yet such an ability to bounce back and stay friends with all her exes. But what is her sex life like now? She's 63 and has been living alone for five years. Has she drawn a line through sex? Certainly not, she says. She is sure she'll continue to meet people and have love affairs, because when you have a lust for life and are warm and welcoming, you attract others. And in the meantime, she's making the most of life's pleasures, such as swimming, letting herself be carried by the water, and caressing herself. "Masturbation is wonderful," she says. "Experiencing self-given pleasure is amazing! I want to give myself that pleasure, so I do! I often say to women who complain about not having sex anymore: you've got hands—use them!"

"When you have a lust for life and are warm and welcoming, you attract others."

Sonia considers herself to be sexual still. She orgasms fantasizing about the bodies of the people she has loved. They are there with her. "Pleasure comes easily." Yes, she says, the fact that she gives time to sexual pleasure, although it is solitary for now, keeps her going, keeps her generous, and keeps love in her heart. "My experience is that it acts like a magnet," she tells me, going on to relate the story of the 30-year-old gay actor she sat next to and chatted to on the bus the day before, who had taken her hand with incredible tenderness and kissed it. That gesture had given her the dose of happiness she needed to see her through the day.

Her girlfriends tell her it's a shame she isn't with anyone and that she should go on a dating site. But Sonia would rather wait for "the magic of an encounter." "I don't see this phase without a partner as permanent," she says. "Anything could happen!"

It's time to wrap up. Sonia tells me she isn't afraid of growing old, and she loves the age spots dotted over the back of her hands. She approaches getting old with confidence and a reliable set of tools: memories, fantasies, and making intimate contact with people. "Life can only get deeper." She's right.

Women living with women

AND WHY NOT? How many 60-something heterosexual women tell me they think about it? It doesn't mean that they're becoming gay but that they are ready to experience erotic intimacy with a woman: to massage and cuddle one another and give each other pleasure.

Véro tells me she shares an apartment with a woman she met at a Californian massage workshop and gets on with very well. They connected over a very modest massage they gave each other one evening. Véro loves the woman's skin. She loves touching it with gentle, sweeping movements. She gets a kick out of helping her unwind. The ability to make someone feel good is what motivates Véro when she gives massages. In theory, you don't become attached to the person you are massaging. But Véro connected with this woman on an intellectual level—they are both psychotherapists and enjoy going to conferences together—as well as on an erotic, playful level. They love spending an evening from time to time taking a bath, then coming up with a host of ways to pleasure each other. And they are never short of ideas!

When I ask Véro if she misses having a man, she is honest enough to say: "Yes, of course I miss it. I love a man's erotic energy, but I don't want it at any cost." So sharing an apartment with a loving girlfriend who she has fun with and gets on well with suits her just fine for now.

Women as initiators

THE TERM "COUGAR" is generally used in a negative sense. It brings to mind older women as sexual predators who pursue virile young men to satisfy their erotic desires. The porn sites dedicated to them merely reinforce that image.

When men are attracted to older women—usually those who are independent with comfortable disposable incomes or pensions—people tend to believe the main reason is their need for financial security. But that is to overlook another cause: the need to be reassured on an emotional level about their identity as a man who can pleasure a woman.

Many single women my age have told me they play a key role in getting their casual lovers' sex lives going again. They say they help these men—who often arrive "broken" by younger women because of their prejudices about male sexual performance—rediscover their self-confidence.

I remember hearing the story of a 45-year-old man who had been happily dating a 70-year-old woman for four years. He acknowledged she no longer had the body of a young girl, but nothing in the world would have made him give up his relationship with that "amazing woman." He valued her experience and her ability to express her desires. "It surprised me that she was so attractive at her age. I felt a little awkward the first time she undressed. But she was so comfortable with her body image and in her skin that my uneasiness soon disappeared." The man confided that he had been suffering from erectile dysfunction when he met her. He had come out of a painful separation with a woman who had constantly belittled and crushed him, and he had lost all his self-confidence. He was genuinely grateful to his older lover for having helped him recover his virility.

It would be wrong to underestimate the role of women in the sexual initiation of men. I've always believed that young men are very lucky if they are introduced to the art of love by older women. Similarly, I think mature women can help men with erection problems get their confidence back.

I've just reread *In Praise of Older Women* by Stephen Vizinczey. This erotic bestseller opens with the advice of Benjamin Franklin: "In all your amours you should prefer old women to young ones ... because they have greater knowledge of the world."[40] A young man called András recounts his first affair with a woman 25 years his senior, Maya. She initiates him into making love and gives him so much self-confidence that he feels he has "the makings of a leader." When they are not castrators, women can give men the feeling they are real men. Vizinczey explains how in the pages of his delightful book. "Maya was teaching me everything there was to know. Yet 'teaching' is the wrong word: she was simply pleasing herself and me [...] She delighted in every motion [...] making love with her was a union, and not the inward masturbation between two strangers in the same bed. 'Watch me now,' she warned me before she came, 'you'll enjoy it.'"

The best way for a woman to give a man confidence is to take care of her own pleasure and involve the man by inviting him to watch her. Which is exactly what Maya does during the sexual union that András speaks of.

My conversations with women who are disappointed by, and in the end bitter about, sex have convinced me that they only have themselves to blame for their frustrations. They haven't chosen to give themselves pleasure and share it with their lovers. Instead they find fault in the lover in question and hold them responsible.

Misunderstandings abound when it comes to men's alleged responsibility for failed sex lives. A 67-year-old man told me that one of his girlfriends had pointed out that his penis was too small. He'd known that for a long time but had discovered it wasn't an obstacle. He knew how to make use of this "disadvantage"; as long as women weren't obsessed with size, he'd learned many ways of connecting with them sexually. He experienced true sexual union with the women who appreciated how wonderful it is to feel a man's penis, in whatever state, at the entrance to her vagina and then to experience the pleasure slowly build.

"The best way for a woman to give a man confidence
is to take care of her own pleasure and involve
the man by inviting him to watch her."

When András ejaculates prematurely, his initiator, Maya, wraps her arms and thighs round him and rolls over without letting him go, ending up on top of him. "You should have a nap," she says, "and let me do all the work."

They make love like that for hours on end. And when he comes inside her, she begs him to stay there because, she says, "I also like it when it becomes small."

• • •

CHAPTER SIX

A different kind of sexuality

Why do some older people still enjoy making love and even say that it's better than before? What is their secret?

• • •

I VENTURED INTO THIS unknown territory of love after turning 60. I had always wondered if the third age could be the age of pleasure and desire, an age we should live fully and consciously in order to serenely take our leave from it as death approached. With the help of experts, I have looked at the psychological and social obstacles to this fulfilment.

I've met many sexagenarians who are experiencing a second adolescence, single women who are doing their best to cope with being alone or who are embracing it joyfully. I've tried to understand what enables couples to stay together, whether or not they make love, and I've entered the relatively unexplored area of those who have given up sex. Now I've come to the heart of the matter: why do some people still enjoy making love as they grow old and go so far as to say that it's even better than before?

This is the secret realm of those who are in love with love and always will be. Some couples are brave enough to say that they continue to have a sex life as they grow older but that it is *completely different*. What exactly are they talking about? What is the nature of this desire that age cannot erase? Their desire for bodily contact, for the sensual feel of skin on skin, for tenderness and the infinite possibilities it creates, now replaces the (in)famous orgasm—the *tyrannical* orgasm that so many younger couples feel pressured to achieve to meet the standards of contemporary society and that ageing men and women are more than happy to escape at long last! Happy, then, are the couples who are able to invent a new kind of sexuality. Not by trying at all costs to keep the weak spark of their existing sexuality alive, with the help of Viagra and sex toys, but by switching to a new eroticism: togetherness, oneness, and sharing a love nest, something you experience when you surrender to each other lovingly and sensually, which can include being physically intimate with each other. Taking intimacy to unlimited depths, as François Jullien might say.

You don't experience real sexual pleasure until you've turned 60

I'M DELIGHTED TO share the wonderful conversation I had with the author and actress Macha Méril.[41] I've always considered her an intelligent, free-spirited woman, and I like the way she discusses her sexuality in her books.[42] She talks about it rationally, humorously, and very openly, giving the impression that she feels perfectly comfortable with the subject. She manages to do something that seems very rare—she discusses sex with *indiscreet discretion*. Apologies for this oxymoron, but I think it suits her perfectly. I also like the way she refers to her vagina as a separate "person," prone to her own insecurities, and, alternately, bursts of enthusiasm that Macha doesn't always understand; a "person" who may occasionally go on strike, when

Macha would really like her to be present and to cooperate, and who doesn't always agree with Macha's choices!

When I read in the media that Macha had just met an 82-year-old man and that they were going to marry, I summoned up the courage to contact her. "Your incredible zest for life and sensuality inspires women of our generation to not give up on love," I wrote, asking her for an interview. She immediately agreed, because this is one of her favorite subjects.

Macha sits opposite me in a short, brightly colored dress and vibrant multi-hued tights. She is bubbly and animated and easily looks ten years younger. She knows it, too. She knows people are astonished when she tells them her age: 73 going on 74! And she hasn't even had cosmetic surgery—just hormone replacement therapy (HRT), which boosts her energy levels and also, as we know, keeps her skin looking good and her joints flexible.[43] It's a treatment she says "all women should have" even though they're now being advised to give it up, for reasons she thinks are hard to justify.

Macha is positively glowing and is in love with the celebrated composer Michel Legrand, aged 82, whom she plans to marry. They first met 40 years ago at a jazz festival in Rio de Janeiro, but they were both married at the time. Although they fell in love, they never acted on it. They reconnected in November 2013, when they were both single, and decided to stay with each other for good this time.

I think she's beautiful and tell her so. "A woman is beautiful when she loves herself," she replies, and "when she loves herself, others find her desirable." It's that simple, she seems to be saying from the outset. How do ageing women see themselves? When you feel good, when you take care of yourself, your health and fitness, when you exercise your mind as well as your muscles and continue to be a loving person who is interested in others, when you're cheerful and curious about everything, then you radiate a kind of positive energy, and it doesn't matter what effects time has had on your body, it is still attractive. Better still. You can't separate the body from the person. It's the person—their charm, spirit, and zest for life—that people find attractive.

Macha: "A woman is beautiful when she loves herself ...
[and] when she loves herself, others find her desirable."

We talk more about this first condition: having a positive self-image. If it's important when we're young, it becomes even more so as we grow older. It is nothing to do with being narcissistic, obsessed with yourself and your appearance. Quite the opposite. A healthy amount of narcissism helps you relate to others. Self-esteem provides a solid base from which to reach out to people or welcome them in.

Macha tells me that she is careful about what she eats and looks after her body "to feel better, stronger, and more sensual"—and because she enjoys it. She keeps fit because "when you grow older, your body deteriorates a bit," but she thinks she has "attractive wrinkles." "Like you!" she says, which makes me feel good.

Macha explains that she is "interested" in her ageing process. "I want to see myself grow older. I'm curious to see what I'll become. Every day is different. When you're loved by someone it's extraordinary—it transforms your face! Haven't you noticed how much younger you look after you've made love?"

She then reminds me that in one of her books, she tells the story of a woman who has just made love with an expert, a ladies' man who constantly has sex with every woman he meets.[44] She asks herself what she's done and, looking in the mirror, is amazed at what she sees. Although she isn't a great beauty, she looks radiant, magnificent. "Don't you find that you become more beautiful during the act of love?"

"If the first condition for remaining interested in and open to love after 60 is having a positive self-image, the second," Macha tells me, "is being able to surrender during love and sex." You need to feel fairly self-assured to give yourself to the other person with confidence. This is when you delve into "the mysterious realm of old-age love"—when you don't have much more to prove, when most of the goals you set yourself are behind you, and you're free at last! Free to be yourself, free with your time, free to choose what you want to do and who you want to do it with. It's why, she continues, "you don't experience real sexual pleasure until you've turned 60."

Before she met Michel, Macha had two or three tumultuous affairs that lasted seven years each. When the most recent one ended, she told herself that she wasn't good at choosing her partners. So be it! She got used to being on her own. In the end, she found that being an independent woman who earned her own living and lived alone wasn't that bad. "I'm sure it's to do with my Marxist past, but I've never had to depend on a man. I think being financially independent is essential for a woman to have a voice. So I was quite well off when we met. He liked that!"

"I don't think we'd have connected if he'd known I was with another man. Or if I'd known he was with another woman. I'm no homewrecker. It would be unthinkable for me to steal a man from another woman. Living with someone is very complicated. You need to leave it up to fate to make sure you're both single."

Macha: "If the first condition for remaining interested in and open to love after 60 is having a positive self-image, the second is being able to surrender during love and sex."

And Michel was, because he had just left his partner—"a harpist who shared his love of music" but clearly nothing more, because the relationship was very stormy, Macha tells me. So he ended it.

How was their reunion? Macha says she was very nervous. She quickly found out that Michel had overcome some serious health issues. They decided to spend a week together. And from the very first evening, she realized they were made for each other. "It was sensational. I was blown away. All my worries disappeared." Their relationship turned out to be easy-going and natural, with a sense of companionship and humor that helped them look beyond the "flaws and the less attractive moments." They laugh a lot, says Macha, who tells me that she likes to laugh, because it opens doors. It reminds you that life is a game you shouldn't take too seriously, while taking it serious-ly—a strange oxymoron!

On the second day, Michel told her, "I'm going to marry you." Macha loved his decisiveness and mascu-linity. "He saw the future of our relationship before I did. He was the first to 'see' it. Isn't that what masculinity is all about? Grabbing hold of a situation and taking charge of it?" I sense Macha feels a lot of admiration for this man who, when they first met, hadn't wanted to "shake up their lives," but who, after seeing her photo on the invitation she sent him for her play, was "able to see the big picture" and get involved with her. "The fact that he had this intu-ition gives me confidence. It allows me to be even more of a woman."

Macha confides that "something incredible" is hap-pening to her. I'd read somewhere that sexual satisfaction increases for women over 50. The female orgasm becomes more intense, apparently, and women who couldn't cli-max before are finally able to. Macha confirms this: "I've never experienced so much pleasure or had such powerful orgasms." She tells me people retort by saying, "Of course, because you've had lots of men!" But it's got nothing to do with how many lovers you've had, she replies. "It's about surrendering! You have to go in with no expectations, so whatever happens exceeds all your expectations. That's the great thing. I've been dressed down plenty of times because of what I write about sexuality, as if I were just playing a game to prove my independence or emancipa-tion. It's not like that at all! I don't give a damn about being emancipated. I'm not taking an exam! It's quite simply that my relationship with pleasure has changed."

But what exactly is this "real sexual pleasure" you only discover after you've turned 60? "It's a *loving* pleasure, because I don't believe in sex without love," Macha continues. "It clearly exists, but this isn't the sexual pleasure you discover after 60. The sexual pleasure I'm talking about involves body, mind, and soul. It's a meeting on the highest level of two kindred spirits who are both equally in love with each other. People often say that in love you must complement each other, but I don't believe it. That may be fine when you just live together, but not when your relationship is an intimate, erotic union. The latter requires you to agree on goals and values and share the same mindset. When there are differences—too many differences—it might be fascinating to begin with, but it quickly stops working!"

"Let's return to this concept of sexual pleasure," I say. "What is it?"

"We're not trying to achieve a goal, such as orgasm, for example. Whether we come or not isn't important. I get irritated with all this talk in the media about the length of a man's penis, his erection, orgasms. Why this obsession? This isn't what sexual pleasure is about at all. There are infinite ways of experiencing sexual pleasure, and some are even more intense than having an orgasm."

Macha then tells me that she and Michel sometimes start making love after a conversation. "A lovely conversation in which we reach the same conclusion and discover new things about each other. I find the words and he seconds everything I say. It's quite extraordinary; we make love by talking, and sex follows on naturally. It's as if we were melting into each other, but not just through sex, through our whole bodies, and through *the idea of making love.*

I've become multi-orgasmic. I come all the time, from start to finish, in waves of pleasure. And it's unlike anything I've experienced before. We go very far."

I attempt an explanation. "What you're saying is that you're so open to love that you make love constantly, whether you're eating a meal or in bed. Everything is eroticized. Is it because you can feel you love each other that you *go very far*?"

Macha Méril's notion of going "very far" reminds me of the "somewhere else" discussed by Jean-Luc Nancy and Adèle Van Reeth in their book on sexual pleasure.[45] "The desire to go out of yourself—is that what you experience?" I ask Macha.

"Your bodies become lighter," she replies. "You escape the concrete, material world. It becomes almost abstract. You're in another universe, and nothing, absolutely nothing, can bring you back to your physical self—neither your sweat nor anything else. You're hyper aware of your bodily state and that of your partner. You're not objectifying your bodies anymore, you're sensing them. You look into each other's eyes, but you're not assessing each other anymore. When you're younger, you assess each other with your gaze because you desperately need reassurance, but not at our age! And it's no longer the case of one night of sex, then another night of sex, in isolation. It's a continuous experience from one time to the next, which I'm very curious about. Rather than being isolated little events, they form a long, amazingly sensual story that twists and turns."

What Macha finds particularly satisfying is the sense that Michel and she are one. "We're two people in one, from the moment we start making love to the moment we stop.

I'm no longer one person—I dive into him and he dives into me. I become part of him. We're a single entity. It's really very, very mysterious! I reach pinnacles of sexual pleasure, and sometimes I feel I'm almost levitating."

Macha then quotes French philosopher Pierre Teilhard de Chardin and his belief that you can glimpse what you might be if you weren't flesh and bones. She concludes: "True sexuality is spiritual. Body and spirit become one! When lovemaking is truly great, no act is more sublime. It's a communion in its truest sense. In my opinion, it's the only communion."

Macha: "And it's no longer the case of one night of sex, then another night of sex … Rather than being isolated little events, they form a long, amazingly sensual story that twists and turns."

Hearing Macha Méril talk about the spiritual dimension of erotic love reminds me of an interview with a woman in Régine Lemoine-Darthois and Élisabeth Weissman's book *Un âge nommé désir* ("An Age Called Desire"): "When I talk about spirituality in a loving relationship, it's when, for example, we are both in a kind of meditative state, motionless, as if we were connected to the universe. It's a state of pure pleasure, but there's no climax, no orgasm, just the joy of being. It's like meeting God himself … everything within us opens up to the other and to the world."[46]

Does Macha know that she's breaking a lot of stereotypes? She paints a picture of the free-spirited, playful, self-aware "new sexuality" that philosopher Robert Mis-rahi spoke of with regard to what we might discover as we grow older. Is it specific to maturity?

"Yes," she replies. "There's a new sense of freedom because you have nothing more to prove to each other. Perhaps this is what maturity brings: having no expectations, no goals, and surrendering yourself with delight. When you're young, the idea of pleasure is unsettling, and you also have certain doubts about yourself and your decisions. Are you living up to others' expectations? Are you sexy enough? Are you a good lover?" Macha tells me about the conversation she recently had with retired French opera singer Natalie Dessay. "Natalie no longer has to achieve the goal of becoming a great singer, and now she sings for pleasure. It's the same kind of thing. I'm not saying that I didn't used to make love for pleasure but that this pleasure was shot through with all kinds of anxieties, whereas now it is pure. It's open to all sorts of possibilities, and I'm extremely curious to discover them."

As I listen to Macha I think about this "openness to new experiences," which is perhaps the only true key to "growing old happily." Is it because there is this "communion of body and soul" between Macha and Michel that they want to marry, and what's more, in church? Macha then tells me she is a non-believer and agnostic but is Russian Orthodox by tradition, a religion characterized by music. The services are composed by great musicians, and when she suggested to Michel that they marry in Alexander Nevsky Cathedral in Paris, she told him, "An Orthodox religious service is like a concert. We get married for the music."

Macha confirms something I already know, which is that in the Russian Orthodox church, you are allowed to make mistakes. You can get married three times. "The second time you can remarry in white. But if it's your third marriage, you do it in black." Since Michel has been divorced twice, he is also able to marry in church but must convert to Russian Orthodoxy, which he has agreed to do out of love for Macha.

Macha: "There's a new sense of freedom because you have nothing more to prove to each other. Perhaps this is what maturity brings: having no expectations, no goals, and surrendering yourself with delight."

"It's a luxury we're allowing ourselves," concludes Macha. They have both decided to get married in a religious ceremony because their marriage is not a social act. They are not getting married for society. They want to tell the world that life is full of surprises and that they have committed to start a new life together and experience everlasting love. "Perhaps we'll discover the true meaning of marriage for older people—a marriage that is unnecessary yet joyful."

Macha is well aware that their marriage bothers some people, in a world where marriage doesn't make much sense anymore, except for young people who want to start a family or gay couples. Theirs is a very unusual marriage, not least because their own children will be requesting the pleasure of their guests' company on the wedding invitations.

"Basically, we're giving form to our desire. Isn't that a great thing to do for two creative people like us?"

A less wild and more complete sex life

YOU MIGHT THINK that only women are able to talk about this "different kind of sexuality" that could "enhance old age," which Robert Misrahi writes about so well. But you'd be wrong. Men can also access it, often thanks to women, as we'll see in the next two accounts.

My friend Régis is a journalist. He's been leading a double life for a long time, and deep down, it suits him. Married with four children and several grandchildren, he has never wanted to jeopardize the family life he's built over the years, because it means a lot to him. But he's a romantic soul, a "romantic by nature," as he puts it. Love vibrates in every fiber of his being, and he can't live without it.

"I've always been a romantic. It's always been important to me. I used to become incandescent with passion and have torrid, tortured love affairs that would always be tinged with anxiety, because I didn't have enough self-confidence. I spent a long time engulfed in the flames of sexual desire, in the lava. It was blistering hot, but over very quickly." Then, at 40, Régis met a sexually experienced woman of the same age. He was not in love with her at all, but she loved him. The relationship lasted five years. "She helped me discover that lovemaking could last for hours, and I think she discovered it herself with me." Régis tells me that this relationship made him more confident. "It calmed me down," he says. Ten years later, he met another woman and fell deeply in love. "When we made love we would look into each other's eyes. I realized that this had never happened to me before. So I discovered this relatively late in life—that feeling of diving into the other person's soul when I penetrate her."

For the first time in his life he tried to be completely honest with his wife, but it sparked a full-blown war at home. "I was crazy enough to try and get my wife and lover to meet each other. Now I realize it was horrendously brutal for them both." Régis had convinced himself that being frank was a sign of maturity, but he became disillusioned because his wife then cheated on him—and this time it was he who couldn't accept it. He realized he couldn't deal with her doing the same to him. "I became terribly jealous. And seriously depressed." By the time he recovered from his depression, with the help of countless psychotherapy sessions and psychotropic drugs, he was 60 and on his knees, with a wife who was thinking of leaving him because she really enjoyed her newfound freedom.

One day she told him that she'd stay but that she didn't want to hear about his affairs with other women. She wasn't in love with him anymore and was no longer interested in sex, but she was fond of him and didn't want to upset the children and grandchildren.

Régis felt like a "complete idiot" and as if he were practically forced to look elsewhere. He makes a point of telling me that he thinks women are often responsible for their husbands' infidelity. "When it's like Siberia in winter, which of you is really the disloyal one? The man who goes elsewhere, or the woman who refuses to make love for years?"

So he started seducing women again and allowing himself to be seduced. When he told them he was married, they would seem rather surprised. "Really? You'd never guess. You don't act like a married man at all."

Régis had several lovers over the next few years, but they all eventually ended their relationship because, he says, "however free-spirited they are, women want to be married." Was he happy with the situation? Not really, he admits, because he let go of some great relationships that weren't given a chance, and because all the lying ended up corroding his relationship with his wife, who he thought he was protecting.

Then, two years ago, he met a woman ten years younger than him and experienced something completely new. "The first time, we spent three days together, but I was at a low ebb and couldn't get it up, so nothing happened. I found it hard to believe she was okay with it. It had happened to me before, of course, and the women had usually been very sensitive, reassuring me that it wasn't a problem, but this was three nights in a row. Three full nights!" The woman didn't understand how he could stay with her three nights in a row without anything happening. She thought he wasn't interested in her. "Then, on the fourth night, I finally managed it!" She became attached to him, and they continued to see each other.

At the end of the first year, a miracle happened. "Suddenly, I saw her. I saw her beauty. Not her objective beauty, but another kind of beauty, the true one—the light shining from her face. It came out of nowhere! It was a shock to the system. In a split second I saw all the problems this moment would lead to. I told myself that I wasn't going to fall back into a full-blown affair. She suddenly became the epitome of the complete woman."

At this point, Régis starts talking in the present tense, and I realize he's experiencing this right now. "Everything she does is exactly what I want. She's perfectly in tune with me, says the perfect thing every time, and makes me feel like a real man. I've never felt such harmony!"

Over the course of a year, it has helped him regain his lost strength. "I can make love several times a day. And it's got nothing to do with the fact I've taken aphrodisiacs and ginseng! It's a spiritual connection. When we see each other, we say how amazing it is! I trust her completely, and she trusts me, and I never have a problem getting an erection anymore. We can be going about our daily business doing a hundred other things and suddenly decide to make love, and it's electrifying! I feel like I'm burning with passion yet completely serene at the same time. I'm living a paradox. When I told one of my female friends I was in a relationship that was totally erotic yet calm at the same time, she replied, 'You must have found your Shakti.'[47] Perhaps she's right. I feel that I've reached the point where my sex life is less wild and more complete. Being this much in tune with someone else and having such a spiritual connection is a new way of loving. After turning 60, the pieces of the 'love puzzle' all fit together and we can go to the next level. It's extraordinary." Except that outside this erotic connection, their daily lives have become hard to deal with.

Like the others, this woman now wants to make plans for the future. But Régis put his cards on the table right from the start by telling her he was married. She responded by saying it wasn't important. "It doesn't matter," she repeated, saying she was prepared to live out the relationship in the present. Then they both started having feelings for each other, and she began to complain that they couldn't build anything together. She said it was becoming "hopeless" and that "it wasn't going anywhere." He confronted her about her desire to build something. "Build what? At our age?" When he was crippled with debt! He simply couldn't see what he could "build" with her.

Régis: "I've reached the point where my sex life
is less wild and more complete. Being this much
in tune with someone else and having such a
spiritual connection is a new way of loving."

"I'm the kind of man who likes to live in the present. Give me a fantastic evening and a night of lovemaking, and I'm satisfied. I'm not looking for anything else."

"So we've reached this amazing level, and that's where we're staying," she replied. "If our love hasn't blown everything else out of the water, it must be because you're pretending ..."

"That's where we disagree. She thinks that everything else should be blown out of the water, that it shouldn't exist. She's a tigress who sometimes causes terrible scenes. She doesn't understand that what we're experiencing is in me, forever. The fact that I won't leave my wife and that I respect the strength of my old relationship is a kind of benchmark, but I can't make her see that. She should understand that it proves I'm faithful to the people and things I care about."

Régis tells me that it's hell at times. He's torn between two women who both want a piece of him and who put him in impossible situations. Since he's a kind of bigamist who seems to care both about his large family and his "Shakti," why doesn't he behave like a "tribal chief"? I ask him. "You could decide to put your foot down and divide your time between both of them, give them boundaries to make them feel secure and stick to them." Régis seems to think this is a good idea, but I don't know if he'll act on it.

His situation is completely different from Macha Méril's. But they do have one thing in common: they have both discovered a different kind of sexuality after 60 that is less wild and more complete.

A shared erotic world

I LOVE MY researcher friend, Folco. He's a true romantic, a handsome man with sensual lips and a masculine gaze that contrasts with his angelic face. Although he's in a long-term relationship and seems firmly attached to the mother of his children, he has always had love affairs with women much younger than him. Why? It's a question I promised myself I'd ask him. A year ago, at a conference, he met a woman called Marie, who is slightly older than him. They've been having a wonderful affair ever since—an affair that has calmed him down, he says.

During their morning seminar they exchanged looks and ideas and were both interested in what the other was saying and thinking. They wanted to see each other again, quickly said so by email, and soon afterwards ended up meeting for coffee quite naturally. Something was going on between them: an obvious mutual attraction, unsettling yet thrilling. She was very charming, and he instantly knew he wanted to go further. They talked a little about their private lives. He'd assumed she was married or in a relationship, but found out she lived alone. So he had to be very clear right away. He wasn't free and wasn't about to be. But he needed passionate love in his life and had always managed to make time for it. He wanted her to understand from the outset that he was full of contradictions and was very complex, but not nasty. Could she accept him as he was?

It was rather a tall order for this 68-year-old single woman, as she'd been looking to meet someone who could offer her companionship, rather than a secret romantic relationship with all its inherent frustrations. Although she would have much preferred a transparent relationship, she was gradually drawn into the affair he suggested, even though it made her anxious since she knew how dangerous it could be to get involved with a man who wasn't free. But her attraction to him was sufficiently powerful and intriguing for her to risk finding out more. No doubt she'd already sensed the erotic potential of their encounter. She wrote to him, saying that she was under no illusion and that it wasn't the first time a chance encounter had put her in this difficult, confusing position—caught between feeling desire and fulfilling it. She said she was confident in her ability to deal with complicated situations and get through them, *to experience them as fully as possible*. She couldn't help herself—she would stay true to her desire and ignore all other contingencies. In short, if she was going to be torn apart, she wanted to do it with her eyes open.

So she followed her desire, placing her faith in him and in the natural course of events. Because it was clear that they quickly felt desire for each other, then love.

When Folco told me this story, I must admit that I didn't think the relationship would last. I thought they'd leave each other. Every time we spoke on the phone, I would ask him how his illicit love affair was going. At first he was afraid of the emotional intensity between them, afraid of getting embroiled in a "folly" that would end with both of them getting hurt. They were managing to see each other quite often and even spending a few days together here and there. He always came away happy, because within the strict confines of their relationship he thought he was doing this woman some good and by extension doing himself some good. It was obviously a great relationship in which eroticism played a central role. He was particularly struck by the way they immediately and quite naturally became intimate with each other. After all, weren't they practically strangers? Now they would spend hours making love with each other, slowly, gently, and sometimes passionately. They were completely focused on each other. I'll confess this fascinated me.

This is why, when I was talking to him one day about my book on love and sex after 60, I asked if he'd agree to be interviewed. As a man who had always been attracted to younger women, what had drawn him to this older lady? I wanted him to tell me in his own words, and for the benefit of my readers, what he was getting out of this romantic relationship.

Why even talk about age? It's trite: as men get older they often lose interest in their partner and turn to younger women for reassurance, because youth is synonymous with sexual power, and younger women offer a narcissistic mirror that validates them. Folco then points out that both sexes engage in this sexual hunt for someone younger. Women of a certain age are attracted to younger men for the same reasons. But they are looked down upon by society, and the fact they are called "cougars" is telling, he says. What we're looking for in a younger partner is to feel young again ourselves. "It's exhilarating," says Folco. "There are moments of intense passion, and you do things you might not have dreamed possible at our age. I've never given up on this passionate intensity, but I'm finding out that I can experience it with a woman who's slightly older than me, and that's new. It's undoubtedly because she *is* young at heart. And that has nothing to do with age."

Perhaps it's this *inner youthfulness* combined with a certain maturity that is attractive. Making love with a woman of her generation means you avoid having to deal with demands you can't meet. Not so much sexual demands, but demands to live together and to have children—things you're no longer interested in when you're 60. Folco knows men his age who have "rebuilt their lives" and have six- or seven-year-old children with a younger woman. "What I see most often in those cases is that, even if they're happy, they're trailing in the wake of their wife's desire, and their lives are geared to that desire. In a way, it's the price they have to pay. Their desire has become a hybrid."

But women who no longer want to have children have different desires and may well have a more open-minded attitude to pleasure, especially if they're not hoping for something specific, such as a new relationship to help them escape their loneliness. If they address their own desires, and, continues Folco, "if they agree to explore their complexities with their partner, then I think you're in an ideal situation. Though it might be rare."

"Women who no longer want to have children have different desires and may well have a more open-minded attitude to pleasure."

Folco thinks he is in this "ideal" erotic situation right now. "I'm touched by the way she uses her romantic intelligence," he tells me. He's met a very sensual woman, and their combined sensuality allows them to endlessly explore their eroticism. "Every time that I've felt I was going further with my own pleasure, it's because she was surrendering to me and giving me the chance to give her pleasure. In short, it's a contradiction: surrendering means giving at the same time as receiving, giving because you receive simultaneously and not successively. You create a kind of delicate balance between the two of you that requires you to be able to let go and paradoxically to 'make sure you do.'"

Folco then uses the metaphor of surfing to describe various aspects of his experience—not only the pleasure he feels at the peak of his own enjoyment, by holding himself back, but also the way he lets himself be guided by Marie's act of surrender, while staying in tune with her. "It's like my senses are heightened, like my entire body is a sensitive instrument that reverberates with each of her body's movements, which I interpret quickly, with the risk that I might make a mistake. Then, each time, I have the pleasure of realizing that I haven't made a mistake and that our pleasure has combined into one, because we've created that pleasure together. What results is one body, *our body*. So, is it our age that allows us to do this? Perhaps a certain kind of sensual sedimentation gives us the confidence to go further—although you have to meet the right person who will let it happen."

Folco thinks you acquire this sensual *density* with age. And age may also make you want to take your time and go more slowly—something you might have denied yourself up to now, because your life was too hectic. Intense passion, emotions, and sensations are therefore not just associated with youth. Folco is realizing this now. What he is going through with Marie is no less intense. Quite the opposite. "It's an overwhelming experience." In fact, concludes Folco, "I think you get better and better at making love as you age, as long as you've always been deeply interested in the experience. It's another way of opening up to another person, being curious about them and needing love. If you don't have that, you can't improve anything. Romantic relationships are profoundly ethical. Bodily intimacy is so arousing that every time you get the chance to make love with someone new for the first time, it's as if you are actually making love for the *very first time*."

Folco tells me he was intimidated the first time they made love. He was afraid his desire would be affected by being with someone new. Would he want her completely, to the end? He feared he'd lose his sex drive and she'd be disappointed. He couldn't be sure on either count. "My penis didn't get very hard. It kept on swelling and deflating. Being with a relative stranger made me full of doubt and uncertainty. What did she expect? Did she want specific things? Did she like my type of virility? Or was she looking for someone a bit rougher? All those ideas and questions were swimming around my head and kept getting in the way, but they were like a transparent net, and I gradually managed to discover her through it. I've forgotten if she came the first time, but I know she liked the gentle way I touched her and liked me kissing her. I felt she was genuinely in tune with me and that she was enjoying it too, which encouraged me— even if for a moment I thought she was a bit 'bossy,' because she immediately asked me *not to move* and declared from the start that she was 'a Tantric woman.'"

"Age may also make you want to take your time and go more slowly—something you might have denied yourself up to now, because your life was too hectic."

"So we started making love slowly," Falco continues. "I entered her gently and stayed in her without moving, then I made a slight rocking motion with my pelvis, and I could tell she liked it. The second time I wasn't afraid anymore, but I was still a bit intimidated. This time I moved more, and she told me she liked that, too." Folco realized that Marie liked all styles of lovemaking. She had no preconceptions. "So I decided to start imagining *our* body. Of course, it wasn't a conscious decision, but I felt this image build inside me as I was desiring her. I quickly realized that she was exceptionally sensual but that she was also a loving woman who wanted and needed to feel permeated by love. I didn't expect that of a woman her age."

Folco thought—and isn't this what paralyzes many men?—that Marie would want certain things and expect him to behave in a particular way. But that's not what happened. She seemed to be open to all possibilities, both on an erotic and an intellectual level. "I've rarely met someone so willing to try new things, yet so deeply attached to her convictions." There's something inspired and determined about this woman, Folco tells me, but she's also free-spirited. "It's the same on the physical level, and I felt that she would follow me wherever I took her."

Will Folco tell me more? I'm fascinated by his story and by this sublime erotic encounter, at an age when many people believe nothing interesting is going to happen to them anymore. I think back to my interview with Macha Méril, who confided that she was discovering uncharted erotic territory in her older years.

Yes, Folco tells me, he thinks Marie has gone further with him than with anyone else. And by allowing him to take her so far, she has opened up a vast world for him. "As I explore her body with my penis, tongue, and hands, I feel her vibrate so intensely that I experience something extraordinary both physically and psychologically. One day I remember feeling like we could go on forever without stopping. Her orgasms just kept on coming one after the other the way jazz musicians blow continuously in their instruments without pausing for breath, so nothing can stop them except the music itself, because it's modulated on their inhalations and exhalations. It was so intense that I was almost scared."

Folco is aware that seeing a woman experience this amount of pleasure gives a man a narcissistic sense of satisfaction, since it proves his potent virility. But what he's describing here goes well beyond that stage or level, to the extent that, while it's a relatively important component of pleasure to begin with, it gradually disappears when you share erotic moments of such intensity.

I think this *shared erotic world* seems to be at the heart of the spiritual aspect of sexual love. "It's no longer about the self: it's about a 'self–other' or an 'other+self,' perhaps an 'other *of* the self,' because you don't fully surrender, but also an 'other *than* the self,' because you go beyond yourself towards the other until you surrender to them almost entirely. It's within these limits, the realm of the 'almost' and 'not quite,' that the magic of pleasure given and received takes place, given because it's received and received because it's given." Folco says he's able to experience this self-abnegation because Marie is completely sincere, and "her enthusiasm is immense, like an invitation to constantly keep going further."

Folco reveals that on several occasions he, too, has reached a point where he's entered an almost mystical, trance-like state. "I understand the meaning of the word *spirituality*, which in this case is the exact opposite of the word sensuality. I'd never made love like that before. Yet sometimes I've been propelled to peaks of sexual pleasure that have bordered on painful. But this experience was totally new. *I endured the pleasure we shared*, the pleasure of giving her almost suffocating pleasure."

As with the Taoist art of loving, Folco notes that he does not ejaculate much. This is new. "But perhaps it takes me somewhere else, even further. However, I've been practicing 'holding back' for a long time now, and it's always given me an enormous amount of pleasure, but with her I don't even need to think about it anymore. Suddenly, I completely focus on her and on her pleasure, and it literally takes me to a higher plane."

Folco's account interests me for two reasons. It's sublime, but it also shows that a woman over 60 can lead a man to peaks of sexual pleasure—perhaps because at her age she can finally experience her sensuality freely, and surrender to it. Folco, who has chalked up a lot of experience with younger women, says he's surprised by Marie. "She expects nothing from her partner: she just expects him. She seems to expect him to be *everything he is*. Maybe she's able to do this because of all the other life experiences she's accumulated. I don't know, but what I do know is that without her willingness to try anything, it wouldn't work. Does your body become like a philosopher when you grow old? Does it have a better idea of what gives it the most pleasure? Maybe, but you still have to listen to it and be open to love for it to happen."

Choosing joy as the fabric of life

HAVING REACHED THIS point in my journey, I wanted to re-read *La joie d'amour* ("The Joy of Love") by Robert Misrahi.[48]

You'll remember I first mentioned Misrahi at the start of this book, because he's an elderly philosopher who speaks from experience. He talks about himself, what he's been through, and what he's going through now at his advanced age.[49] I believe that the opinions of a very old man on love and desire are particularly valuable. The joy of love is possible, challenging, even desirable, he asserts, for everyone who is moving into the mature stages of love. It is, for him, "one of the fundamental concerns" of his philosophy and life. Choosing joy as the fabric of life is preferable to any other form of existence.

Misrahi is well aware of the obstacles to "the joy of love," which he skillfully analyzes, and which he believes arise from the institution of monogamy (the weariness that causes love to end; the domination of one by the other; possessiveness and its corollary, jealousy; misunderstanding and betrayal). In light of all this, he also shows us how, as human beings blessed with freedom and the power of reflection, we can overcome these obstacles, to "invent"— the word comes up frequently—new paths.[50]

> "Choosing joy as the fabric of life is preferable to any other form of existence."

He expresses his disgust at the kind of sexuality that is an end to itself: "Nights of pure sexual bingeing, soulless orgies, consumerist swinging, the accumulation of sexual conquests, open relationships."[51] In short, a sexuality that "at best makes us jaded and bored, and at worst makes us anguished by the absurdity and loneliness we feel at the evident lack of love."[52] He knows that time brutally attacks love, that it often damages and destroys it, and that habit kills it. He knows that ageing changes things and that you become jaded after a while. However, he still believes love is the only thing that is really worth experiencing, and despite all the catastrophes and failures we suffer, he is convinced there are solutions to help love achieve its goal: joy and fulfilment. "Ways of being inventive" are possible at any age. And he deserves to be taken seriously, because he is a very old man who speaks from experience.

Desire can hit us out of nowhere, but love must be built, and *the joy of love is a choice.* We must also want it—want joy, want sexual pleasure, want freedom. The three terms are intimately entwined in this erotic happiness, which, as you'll remember, Misrahi believes could contribute to "enhancing old age," and which concerns "the physical body, made of flesh, desire, emotions, pleasures, quivers, and caresses."[53]

"Desire can hit us out of nowhere, but love must be built, and *the joy of love is a choice.*"

Misrahi gives us ways to achieve this and tells us what to do with our body and mind to ensure that joy remains. The desire for sexual pleasure implies a *conversion.* This philosophical term has nothing to do with religious conversion. It's a term Misrahi is fond of, and it refers to the period of reflection every person blessed with freedom is called on to undertake if they want to "build" a loving relationship. *Conversion* describes the inner psychological work couples need to do to attain "high love."

Reflecting on two of love's major pitfalls—jealousy and possessiveness—will lead, if we want it to, to a different notion of love, in which each partner respects the other's freedom and will inevitably gain a better understanding of *who* the other person is.

Misrahi also examines another obstacle to love: "lack of understanding" or "misunderstanding." We think we love someone but realize over time that we don't know them at all. We don't know *who* they really are. We build a life together on a foundation that's somehow rotten. Or else our partner doesn't know us—perhaps because we haven't allowed them into our intimacy. They criticize and blame us. Our self-esteem is violated and trampled on. Sooner or later, if we're in a relationship, we're bound to face the anthropological problem that is monogamy and the sexual exclusivity attached to it. How do we remain faithful to one person our whole life? "Not all people are willing or able to accept it for a long time."[54] Transgression, if it is a pleasure, usually leads to lies and deceit. The gap between betrayer and betrayed widens. If the one being deceived experiences this betrayal as a "symbolic assassination," the deceiver, whose motives for the transgression are not understood, experiences a sort of "symbolic annihilation" of the core of his or her being. Silence and lack of understanding eventually lead to a separation of minds, Misrahi tells us, and the most likely result is the failure of the loving partnership.[55] The strength of their commitment to each other is called into question.

So what should we do? The solution to all these problems doesn't lie in institutional polygamy, which, as

Misrahi proves, causes as much suffering as monogamy, nor in open relationships or casual sex, which don't involve love, but in types of love that respect the person or people who are loved. Of these types of love, exclusive, reciprocal, and *faithful* love is extremely rare, he admits. Faithful love implies that "each person commits to learning more about the other's body and personality in an ongoing process"; the couple mutually decides to "develop their love, intimacy, and tenderness in the long term. In this kind of relationship, the goal is to continually deepen their intimate knowledge of each other and to accept their personality and its limitations."

The other type of love that may avoid the kind of suffering that can spell the end of a relationship is *multiple love*, the possibility of loving several people at the same time, freely and peacefully. What does he mean by that? We've seen that Misrahi condemns open relationships, and we know that the expression "multiple love" has little to do with orgies and swinging or even the polyamory movement, which argues for transparency in multiple relationships.[56] "Each person says to the other, 'We love each other and form a precious unit together; but we are both free-thinking human beings who are completely unfettered by tradition or moralism, and by offering to tell each other about our affairs, we embody a new morality of freedom and responsibility.'"[57] So there is no betrayal or deceit. This moral code of transparency would be welcome, Misrahi tells us, if it saved the life of a loving relationship by overcoming the issue of jealousy. But things don't work that way.

By analyzing *She Came to Stay* by Simone de Beauvoir, a proponent of this theory of transparency, Misrahi clearly shows us that we have a long way to go. When Xavière suddenly bursts into Pierre's life, Françoise is terribly hurt. After all—says Misrahi—when someone reveals a truth to their partner that suggests that their relationship has become inadequate and that their partner is no longer erotically or emotionally attractive enough to fulfil their desire, isn't this a little sadistic? Or thoughtless, at the very least? Does true love still exist between them? Doesn't transparency kill love, even when it is agreed on in advance and insisted upon by both partners?

We read on in suspense. Misrahi obviously believes that the joy of love—a fulfilling, intense joy he describes as "the highest justification for existence"—does not require exclusivity. A man or woman may experience joy with their partner yet at the same time experience intense joy in a relationship with a third person. It's not a utopia, he says. It's a "reality of human existence." But it's a reality that is not necessarily easy to live with.

"Doesn't transparency kill love, even when it is agreed on in advance and insisted upon by both partners?"

There are two possible ways forward, he says. One, *philosophical love*, which is also rare because it implies a mutual respect for each other's freedom and independence within the relationship, and the implicit acceptance that one or both partners may have another loving relationship. Or two, *secret love*, which is much more common but not without its risks or suffering, even if this suffering is far different from the suffering described earlier that leads to the end of a loving relationship.

The ethics of secrecy involve frustrations and constraints. When these frustrations and constraints are freely agreed to by both members of the relationship, their love becomes deeper, and the suffering they cause is "a constituent of love." The ethics of secrecy are challenging for those who freely decide not to give up any of their loving relationships and not to let a moral sense of duty or sacrifice stop them from giving in to their desire. While they refuse to be "taken hostage" by their partner or to sacrifice a new love on the altar of duty, they are nonetheless careful not to hurt the person they are tied to through "an old love." "Respecting and keeping alive the old joy of love do not have to exclude entering into a new relationship and a special love."[58]

Maintaining two loving relationships at the same time and simultaneously experiencing joy and responsibility is certainly challenging, as is pursuing your own fulfilment within a new love affair and "existentially protecting the health and serenity of the person you have loved the longest."[59] But it is possible, and many manage to do it, as long as they are capable of being both open-minded and generous.

But the ethics of secrecy may be even more challenging for those outside the existing relationship. The ethics imply a high degree of evolved, progressive thinking that is far removed from the desire to possess the other. The third party must accept that the man or woman they love is committed to *not hurting* their life partner and therefore accept that they will conduct their love affair in a discreet location, see each other intermittently, and not share a social life. "You can't inflict this level of freedom on someone who hasn't gone through their own *conversion*, because it would have the same effect on them as drinking too much alcohol," comments French philosopher Michel Onfray in the preface to Misrahi's book.[60] The spouse must be protected, as they may be overcome with abandonment anxiety or be unable to contemplate sharing their partner with someone else.

Admittedly, you need to be very generous and loving to freely agree to enter into a "discreet loving relationship." But it is feasible, if you believe you are genuinely loved and if you and your lover have developed mutual trust. "Discreet love is not doomed to fail if it is motivated and sustained by a *deep understanding of the challenges of love*." In other words, if two lovers give themselves fully to each other and are unreservedly there for each other whenever they are together, love can take them higher. They know that the existence of a third person, who they are anxious not to hurt or leave, takes nothing away from the sexual pleasure they experience with each other. They know that there is no need to compare the old love with the new one. All they represent to each other, the way they engage their bodies and minds in the relationship, belongs to a unique and separate world. This is why, affirms Misrahi, the ethics of secrecy, pleasure, and responsibility, whose primary concern is to avoid unnecessary suffering, have nothing in common with lies or betrayal.

Discreet love can be a high form of love, a "successful love." Something that is unable to flourish in our daily lives or social lives can flourish in a "secret garden," away from provocations and jealousy. We know how much these moments of secret intimacy strengthen the connection and how much consensual suffering brings lovers closer together. Discreet love can be long-lasting, says Misrahi. It may be equally as fulfilling as faithful love, "provided that the love affair is conducted in such a way that it does not bring about suffering and ruin around it."

The ethics of secrecy

THINKING ABOUT THE ethics of secrecy made me want to meet Marie, Folco's partner.

I sit opposite her at a table in a bistro and look at her. She's certainly attractive. Folco is right—she's a beautiful woman who looks very young for her age and wears her wrinkles well. I'm especially struck by her soft voice and the slow rhythm of her speech. There is a calm, sensual aura about her.

How should I approach this woman, who I've only just met, about the most intimate aspects of her relationship with Folco, a man who's in love with being in love?

I tell her how moved I was by the way "her man" spoke to me about their relationship, but I also admit to being confused. How does she cope with having a hidden, secret relationship with a man who is not "free," when she is and lives alone? How does she manage not to get frustrated?

"Because I love him and have never had an erotic relationship as wonderful as this," she instantly fires back. Of course, it's not easy. She promised herself never to get involved in a "backstreet" relationship, as she calls it, because she was aware of the pitfalls. But when she met this alluring man with his bright, intelligent eyes and sensual lips, she felt an irresistible attraction to him. And she told herself, "Just go for it and see what happens!" She knew she was being impulsive but also knew that she wouldn't let anyone lead her where she didn't want to go. Since then, the path they have taken together has opened up so many new horizons, emotions, and sensations that she doesn't regret following him in the slightest. It was a risk, but a risk worth taking.

She has her low points, of course. They've gone through long periods of absence during the summer and Christmas holidays. She misses him, and it's painful. But he's asked her not to hide it, and that's surprised her. So she talks to him about it. She now realizes he's not afraid of hearing about it, because instead of withdrawing and feeling guilty, he always consoles her in an amazingly sensitive way. His words prove that he loves and cares about her. She believes he is sincere. So rather than brooding about it and getting caught up in negative thought patterns, such as, "If he really loved me, he'd leave his wife and choose me"—which are actually rather clichéd ways of thinking—she dispels any such thoughts from her mind. Instead, she thinks about the world she is exploring with him, and the unparalleled erotic and sensual connection they enjoy.

It's true that they don't see each other much, but when they do they always have an amazing time. Her best friend, who she often confides in, tells Marie that she gets the best of all worlds. Marie agrees, and this is yet another paradox. Although Folco is unavailable socially, this doesn't prevent him from being fully present and completely engaging his body and soul in their intimate encounters.

I would like to know what is so new, at her age, about her experience with this exceptional lover. Marie describes herself as a cerebral woman. She has made love a lot in her life, but on a very intellectual level. She used to like it fast. She liked men to make her come quickly, press themselves against her, hold her tight, not move, and wait for the waves of pleasure to build until she reached orgasm, which was very powerful. She knew her body well and knew what to do to climax quickly. Now that she's older, pleasure builds more slowly. With Folco, she's experienced surrender. She doesn't try to achieve the same things she used to do. She's discovering a sensuality she never imagined and surrenders to Folco's hands, mouth, and body. He takes her to places she didn't know existed, and she experiences new sexual pleasures that are very intimate. She doesn't want to go into detail, but I get the feeling she has opened doors for Folco that she has never opened for anyone before.

"Folco has no barriers. I've never had a lover as inventive, as in tune with my body, or as gentle as he is. I believe he loves my body, and that's very important to me, because my body isn't so young anymore. But I think that beyond my body's sensual response—and doubtless my soft skin and the way I give myself to him—he loves *me*, the person I am. I feel the same way. I love his deep, sensual, erotic voice. I love how he holds me and penetrates me, the gentle way he explores my body and gives me pleasure. I am penetrated by *him—by all of him*. So I absolutely cherish him as a person, deeply and forever. He holds a very special place in my heart, and I feel I *belong to him*."

Marie and Folco make love for entire afternoons, stopping to drink tea and tell each other stories, then resuming again with even more gusto. Their desire is constantly rekindled, something she has never experienced before. "One of the things I've discovered is the incredible pleasure of feeling his skin against mine when we're naked. Every time it's like the first time! Before him, I didn't really appreciate this."

This near-permanent state of desire continues after he leaves. They are able to maintain it through their almost daily correspondence, she tells me. "He has his own special way of maintaining our desire for each other and of making me feel that I'm important to him. This helps me deal with his physical absence. In fact, as frustrating as it is, this love does me a power of good because it makes me feel like a real woman. What I like about my life right now is this sensual surrender to him."

After Macha Méril, Marie is the second person I've met who says she's now, in her older years, experiencing sexual pleasure that is infinitely longer and more satisfying than the pleasure she used to experience when she was younger. She's the second person who has told me that for her, making love doesn't just mean intercourse. With Folco, Marie "makes love all the time." Their conversations and pleasures are endless and limitless. "I love the confidence with which we whisper serious things to each other, the confidence that has developed between us," she confides.

We talk for over an hour and bond with each other, woman to woman. I feel able to ask her more about what she calls her "exquisite moments." "One night I pulled him against me and asked him to stay still with his genitals touching mine. I asked him to open his eyes and look at me, then we kissed languorously while remaining still. There was a sense of gravity in our embrace that I'll never forget. Our whole beings connected. I felt his penis attracted to me like a magnet, but he didn't move. There was an extraordinary intensity between us. It was as if his soul were enveloping my body. He couldn't believe it. Me neither. Then he was inside me and we were vibrating, still motionless. Waves of pleasure began to build in me, and I felt like I was winding myself around him like a vine, still without moving. It was simply overwhelming. I was suddenly hit by an explosion of pleasure like nothing I'd ever experienced before. And I burst into tears. Tears of emotion—joy and gratitude."

"Making love doesn't just mean intercourse."

Marie tells me that Folco is more than a lover to her. He is the man with whom, and through whom, they both explore the mystery of two bodies that love each other, the mystery of a love that makes something rigid and hard explode within them and forces the light to come in.

"My favorite time is the moment after we've made love," continues Marie. "When our bodies haven't yet separated. When they are indistinguishable for a few seconds. Folco calls it 'our body.' Before, when we were making love, our bodies were separate from each other. He is the penetrating force, and I am a valley that welcomes him and that he ploughs and harvests. He digs deep into me, and I dig deep into myself. Our bodies work at achieving sexual pleasure. And then, when we orgasm, that burning fuse of desire vanishes into thin air. We experience a lightening, a completely new feeling of lightness. I remember reading somewhere that love begins after making love. It's after making love that a woman knows whether the man who has made love to her genuinely loves her. Some men go to sleep and others quickly get wrapped up in their anxieties again. They ruin the love and don't realize the harm they're doing."

So Marie and her "virile angel," as she likes to call him (because, she tells me, there is a physical/metaphysical side to their relationship), proceed like tightrope walkers on a wire. Marie has decided to love their "secret love" and protect it as best she can. It is part of them.

"We have a very deep connection. It's as if we knew each other's essence. I think we are moving forward confidently."

Listening to Marie, I think these two people are living by the ethics of secrecy that Misrahi talks about. It's challenging but possible, and many succeed in it—even if it sometimes takes a lifetime to get there.

Folco and Marie have both agreed to conduct their love affair away from provocations and jealousy, to avoid causing suffering around them. And this works because they love each other and give themselves unreservedly to each other when they are together. The existence of Folco's partner does not detract in any way from the sexual pleasure that he and Marie experience with each other. There is no need to compare them, because for Folco, they each represent a unique and separate world.

They seem to follow the ethics of sexual pleasure and responsibility advocated by Misrahi. And this is why the love that flourishes in their "secret garden" is perceived by Marie as a "high form of love." If they both feel that something is missing, it's a consensual form of suffering that, far from driving them apart, brings them closer together. This is why Marie is confident that their discreet love will stand the test of time.

In search of a new harmony

I'D LIKE TO introduce Philippe, a 68-year-old man who has had a successful career in publishing and is the father of several adult children with his wife, Sophie, who is ten years his junior. He immediately comes across as a man who has always enjoyed making love and whose desire to seduce his wife has not diminished over the years. He still likes feeling aroused by her. In short, they were a couple of youthful almost-sexagenarians with strong desires—until one day, after Philippe turned 60, he felt his passion wane and a jaded feeling creep over him, which made him anxious. Sophie, a doctor, had heard about a little-known sexual practice from India called Tantra, taught by therapists to couples who wanted to "reach a higher state" and find "a new harmony."[61] Philippe agreed to try it, mainly out of curiosity, and together they discovered this different approach to eroticism—different from what they had been practicing together, at least. They were not disappointed. Better still, Philippe tells me that the way they make love has changed and that he is amazed at what he has discovered.

I'm curious, too, and ask him about it. What is Tantra? What was the training like? What did he get out of it?

I then learn that it is an ancient practice that originated in the Indus Valley around five thousand years ago. The men and women made love not only to procreate but also to attain an almost mystical form of ecstasy. They made love very slowly, pausing regularly then resuming, combining the exchange of their breath and skin to create a surge of sexual energy—Kundalini—that traveled up the spine to the top of the head. The goal was to achieve union with the divine and mystical ecstasy, and the sex they practiced focused more on vibration and sensuality than the genitals themselves.

Philippe said very little about the training itself, citing the confidentiality agreement he was asked to commit to. All I learned is that the techniques and exercises were taught in a group, but that each couple practiced them alone at home. No one engaged in the sex act in the training center itself, and this ethos was respected and guaranteed by a couple of highly professional, competent facilitators.

Intrigued, I ask him if group courses like this have an element of pornography and swinging about them. Nothing of the sort, he replies. Tantra is a sacred and spiritual approach to sexuality. You are taught breathing and visualization techniques that help you become aware of the surge in sexual energy within your body. Participants may also refuse to take part in a ritual or exercise. The teaching of Tantra is based on mutual respect.

So what did he discover? Having become anxious, like all men his age, about the future of his sexuality, and aware that his body was ageing sexually, Philippe came away from the course feeling relieved. He discovered that sexuality is not just about the genitals but about vibration, and

that you can experience infinite pleasure and even a powerful orgasm without an erection. "It's incredibly liberating
for a man," he tells me. "After all, when you grow older
you can't get hard as often, as much, or for as long, and
although Tantra hasn't improved that side of things, I've
found out something else—that there's more to life than
getting an erection! In particular, I've realized that I can
desire Sophie in other ways, not just sexually. I desire her
presence, her touch, being with her, feeling her skin, being
felt by her, but we're not obsessed with sexual intercourse."

This discovery has ultimately strengthened their relationship. However, others end up leaving each other after
a course in Tantra, because this aspect of sexuality makes
people face up to a different question: do they love their
husband, wife, or partner? Do they feel good with them?
Do they love being with them? Some couples leave each
other and others get together. And these new couples then
start off with a foundation that's much stronger and more
authentic, because Tantra can be practiced throughout
your life, even at 80, which is good news for all.

CHAPTER SEVEN

• • •

Other erotic ways

What is slow sex and what does it involve?
Are orgasms necessary? What if the answer
to sexual fulfilment is to make less of it?

* * *

"I'm only just beginning to understand their erotic rites,
the process of assimilation by which the man comes to
identify himself, even in his sensations, as one with
the woman he is taking, and to imagine he is her while
remaining himself."

André Malraux, *The Royal Way*[62]

Making love slowly

THE MEN AND women who have taken part in my research
have all confirmed one thing: the way they have sex has
changed. It has become more sensual and tender, and
slower. It has become "different."

I'm not saying that young people don't explore the "slow
sex" trend. I'm saying that older people adopt it by force
of circumstance.

Ageing men who continue to have desires and make
love have completely changed their attitudes towards their
penises. They have finally understood what sex therapists
and women have said all along: size almost doesn't matter!
They have distanced themselves, with a wry smile, from

the image of the super-virile man that haunts the minds of so many men, and from the temptation to take the little blue pill that's supposed to make their penises as hard as steel whenever and wherever they take it.

So the older generation is encouraged to forget about performance. They no longer see orgasms as the be-all and end-all. They have also discovered that by letting their bodies *do their thing*, and by ceasing to be obsessed with erections and climaxing, they become much more present in their intimate encounters. You could say they make love with heightened awareness.

Many books extolling slow sex have come out recently. They all say pretty much the same thing: we must shift from "faster, harder" to exploring something else—namely, a slow kind of sexuality that has been a key practice for millennia in countries such as China and India.

What does this new, Eastern-inspired sexuality involve? Taking your time and forgetting the destination. It's the erotic journey that counts. And it's a sensual one. Skin is equipped with numerous touch sensors. Why not take the time to slowly awaken all the body's erogenous zones and caress them in every way possible? If you make the journey with full awareness, if you are completely present in what you feel, then you are also completely present with your partner and can achieve an unparalleled feeling of erotic union.

Tantric women

I WAS REALLY intrigued by what Philippe had told me about his Tantra course, so I decided to go and find out about it for myself. I could have just read books on the subject, but I thought it would be best to experience it first-hand. So I enrolled in a course called "The Tantric Woman," which I'll try to summarize for you now.[63] I chose a women-only course, because I was scared of being alone in a mixed-sex group for my first experience and I was keen to understand the mysteries of Tantra in a relaxed setting.

The venue is mesmerizing. Located at the foot of Pic Saint-Loup mountain in the Cevennes, the Hameau de l'Étoile hosts personal development workshops in a calm, bucolic setting. I flew out this morning, rented a car, and arrived in brilliant, feel-good sunshine. I'm lodged in a *cassine*, a very comfortable wooden chalet nestling among the trees. I'm rather apprehensive, because even though I'm not quite sure what to expect, I know it's going to be an intimate adventure.

I also wonder what has motivated 40 women aged between 25 and 68 to come on this kind of course. I discover that it has attracted all sorts: unhappy women who I consider very brave to throw themselves in at the deep end like this; unsatisfied or frigid women sent there by an inspired sex therapist; women who have already begun "Tantric self-analysis" and wish to pursue it further; women in failing relationships who have decided to face up to their responsibilities; and, among the older members of the group, women who want to reach a new, more spiritual, and more meditative level of sexuality. What most of them have in common is a great deal of curiosity and a very strong desire for sexual experimentation. They want to explore new territories in their sexuality. I, too, am motivated by curiosity. Although I think I've had a fairly satisfying love and sex life, I believe I have new territories to explore and new sensations and emotions to experience. At my age, I also need to find out what my erotic potential is.

The aim of the course is clear: to help women abandon the conventions that cause them stress and put pressure on them. These days, a fulfilling sex life is an aspect of personal success. The mantra seems to be: "Have as many orgasms as you can, and you'll be happy!"

Women wonder, "Am I normal if I don't have orgasms or if I have fantasies?" Sexuality is often experienced as something complicated, and they find plenty of excuses not to make love, from tiredness and the children to pregnancy. At the same time, women feel that something is lacking, and this is extremely frustrating. Many are confused: should they trust their feelings, or should they rely on what is said in surveys and women's magazines?

The first convention they must give up is the belief that orgasms are compulsory. I learn that only a third of women regularly have orgasms. Does that mean that the remaining two-thirds don't climax?

The aim of this four-day Tantric journey is to help us better connect with our bodies. To hell with performance, to hell with the pressure to orgasm!

It's a very strange experience finding myself in a big room known as the "temple of women" with some 40 other women, all younger than me and all here to uncover the mysteries of Tantra!

Sitting in a circle in the "temple," which is decorated with rather kitsch representations of Shakti and Shiva and brightly colored fabrics,[64] we are asked to introduce ourselves by stating our first names and sexual orientation. Apart from two or three bisexuals, most of the women say they are heterosexual. When it's my turn, I just say, "I like making love with a man."

I learn that there are two ways of Tantra. One way is letting go and surrendering to your sexual organs; the other is trying to reach ecstasy in stages by increasing your sexual energy—Kundalini—chakra by chakra through visualization and breathing techniques.[65]

"To hell with performance, to hell with pressure to orgasm!"

We are promised a beautiful journey into femininity and the secrets of the female body. I have to overcome my modesty when I see my "sisters" strip naked one after the other during a frenzied dance. However comfortable I am with my body, deciding to undress in front of all these women is not easy. I eventually realize it's a liberating experience. There we all are in a circle—fat women, thin women, those with very bushy pubic hair, those with almost no pubic hair, those who are visibly uncomfortable, and those who look quite at home. We laugh a lot, and being naked brings us closer together. I feel like I'm taking part in some kind of mysterious ancient ritual.

One part of the course gives women the opportunity to explore what is preventing them from having a fulfilling sex life. I find this section rather boring, as I've been familiar with this aspect of psychological analysis for a long time. But I admire the tact and professionalism with which the facilitator leads the discussion. We cover everything: the impact of how sexuality is portrayed from one generation to the next, the influence of childhood wounds, rape, abuse, lack of respect by men, and having too idealized a vision of love.

Another part of the course is devoted to the gentle, intimate exploration of our bodies and genitals, because the better you know yourself, the better you know who you are when you give yourself to another person. "When constructing your femininity and sexual fulfilment, the way you experience your genitals is important. That doesn't mean just knowing they are there and where they are located, but being familiar with them, investigating them, discovering them, looking at them, admiring them, and welcoming them." [66] A number of very intimate rituals are suggested, and each takes place in a very controlled way with the greatest respect for everyone there.

"The better you know yourself, the better you know who you are when you give yourself to another person."

There is much talk of surrendering and relaxing, learning about intimate communication, and letting the genitals perform on their own. This last point is definitely the most difficult. Women are often too much in control to achieve orgasm; they almost reach the peak, but then fall back down again.

At one of the meals we have outside under the trees, I find myself sitting next to a woman who is younger than me, with lots of experience of Tantra. She helps me understand what lies at the heart of this sexual yoga. "The pursuit of sexual arousal prevents you from accessing a very sub-tle energy—an incredible pleasure that only comes when you stop trying to achieve it," she tells me. "Men believe," she continues, "that they must maintain pressure on their penises by repeatedly moving them back and forth to keep them erect. They are wrong. They refuse to believe that they can continue to have a hard-on even when they relax. In actual fact, the penis stays erect all by itself if it's drawn up inside a woman who desires him. Her genitals are like a magnet. They pull the man inside her. And if she's in that erotic state of magnetism, the man just needs to pene-trate her very gently and slowly for the spark of orgasm to be ignited."

Over the four days we take part in various meditation sessions, during which we increase our energy very lan-guidly and sensually as we move our pelvises in time with our breathing, contract our perinea (a crucial skill to learn), and create mental pictures.

We practice "reverse breathing" and the "wave" in a position you see all the time in images illustrating Tantric sex: the man sits in the half-lotus posture and the woman sits astride him, facing him, with her legs wrapped around him, so that their genitals are in contact. It's a posture that creates a deep sense of intimacy. With their mouths touch-ing, one of the lovers inhales slowly while the other exhales so they are breathing each other's air. After a few minutes, the breathing automatically becomes synchronized, and you start to imagine your breath descending down into your partner's genitals as they let your breath penetrate them. It is extremely erotic. Each of these experiences is followed by much-needed discussion time.

I come away from the course feeling a huge amount of affection for the tribe of women I've met, and I'm convinced that every young woman would benefit from learning about sexual yoga if she wants to achieve a developed and fulfilling sex life. She would know herself better and could guide her partner as a result. It would see her through life and the highs and lows of her physical changes.

A stone's throw from the women's workshops, a group of around 40 men were also learning about more aware sex.[67] By the look on their beaming, friendly faces, which I glimpsed now and again, it was clearly doing them a world of good, too.

Genitals can make love all by themselves

WHEN I RETURN home, I start reading some of the books the course leaders have recommended. The first is by Barry Long, a late Australian Tantric master who claimed, in the tradition of many before him, that sex is a gateway to the divine.[68] Once I get past the slightly pretentious tone of the author, who talks of his contemporaries as simple-minded materialists of love, I discover some very compelling ideas. *Genitals can make love all by themselves*, Long says. Just let them get on with it; don't impose anything learned or artificial on them. They attract each other like magnets. All lovers have to do is consciously occupy the part of the body where they experience pleasure.

The key thing is to be present in what is happening. Scenes and images from elsewhere, including from the past, and fantasies of all kinds, will prevent lovers from being present in what is taking place between their connected sexual organs. The woman must not do anything she has learned with other lovers or gained by reading or watching films. The lovers must make love as if it were the first time.

"The key thing is to be present in what is happening."

Love should be made very slowly, very gently, and in a loving way, each lover in tune with their own and their partner's genitals. This kind of union has nothing to do with what Barry Long criticizes as consummatory sex, which is when couples frantically pursue orgasms. As I read the book, I think about all those over-60s looking for a new kind of sexuality.

What about men who can't get an erection or can't get fully hard? "The penis can be helped into the partner's vagina," Long writes. "Put the soft penis into the entrance of the vagina. Wait patiently. If there is enough love between them, it will be sufficiently erect to enter her. Or the man should lie down beside her and wait until the love flows. The penis mustn't be handled with haste or force. Once inside, the penis will swell or have a full erection."[69]

The orgasm is part of the act of love, but it comes when it comes, and if it comes, it comes on its own, not because we want it to or we make it happen. "It is not the goal."[70] The goal is to achieve the incredible pleasure of genitals in close contact, left to perform on their own. If this happens, making love can go on and on, "until at last, perhaps hours later, the man ejaculates naturally and consciously.

Or they separate and make love again a few hours later."[71] I am reminded of the couples who told me they make love for hours, over and over again, without tiring.

Barry Long concludes by saying: "Your body doesn't need to learn how to make love. It makes love naturally when given the chance. But your attachment to past experiences creates an obstacle."[72] All that lovers need to do is be psychologically and spiritually present during the act of love, by becoming aware. "Make love for love, not for yourself."[73] This kind of sexuality, in which lovers are "present during the act of love," is sacred. The *yoni* and *lingam* become "spiritual organs."[74]

Erotic retreats

A NEW PHENOMENON has arrived in Europe from California: "erotic retreats."[75] These residential courses, generally inspired by Tantra or Taoism, offer couples in difficulty guidance towards a new art of loving. They are encouraged to let love happen and to give up climax-oriented sex and conventional expectations. This isn't an easy approach to take in modern society, where we all want to take control and master everything. Learning to relax and not obsess about being aroused or climaxing seems to put many people at ease, especially women. Couples who do this stand a better chance of lasting and growing old with each other.

In a book I really enjoyed, *Laisser faire l'amour: un chemin surprenant vers la lenteur sexuelle* ("Let Love Happen: an amazing path to slow sex"), Stephen Vasey invites couples to get out of their lovemaking rut by spending intimate time together, kissing and caressing, but consciously deciding not to make any effort to reach orgasm.[76] Leaving the way open to the unknown will surprise you, he says. You will discover new sensations and pleasures, and they will feel amazing. And if you finally reach orgasm without trying, then all the better, because it is often much more intense.

You can turn this prolonged erotic time into a ritual by creating a lovely atmosphere with candles, incense, and slow, sensual music. It can be punctuated with breaks: taking a bath or shower together, dancing naked, drinking a glass of champagne, or giving each other a massage. You'll discover wonderful sensitivity points hidden all over the body, "in our hollows, folds and recesses, and in and around our orifices."

What if the answer to sexual fulfilment was to make less of it? Stephen Vasey describes what he experienced while his partner was lying on top him after they'd made love. "I was bearing all her weight, and it felt good. Naked, comfortable, and in love, there was nothing for us to do, nowhere to go, except relax together in the glow of the blaze of joy we had just experienced. In this moment of communion, I felt in my body a sense of infinite welcome. Sometimes we breathed in unison, sometimes in sync and sometimes in alternation. It was harmonious, immense, oceanic."

Tiresias's Journey

AS FRANÇOIS PARPAIX has observed, having a satisfying sex life as you grow older requires a sort of energy reversal: women must be more yang and take more erotic initiative;

men must accept their yin side, learn to be receptive, and to *let love happen.*

These days we all know we have both feminine and masculine sides. How can you switch roles and learn to play with both qualities? "Sometimes I take a back seat in an encounter. At other times, I'm the one who initiates, who suggests, who surprises, who takes my partner on a (little) adventure," Vasey writes.

"Women must be more yang and take more erotic initiative; men must accept their yin side, learn to be receptive, and to *let love happen.*"

The criticism often made of Tantra is that it places too much emphasis on the feminine. And that's true. But in an erotic world still very much oriented towards male and yang values (performance, efficiency, initiative), don't we need to inject a little femininity and yin (receptiveness, expectation, welcome) in order to create harmony in our relationships?

Yet many men resist making that change. And when they start to feel less virile as they grow older, they prefer giving up sex rather than exploring something else. Jacques Ferber, author of *L'amant tantrique* ("The Tantric Lover") is well versed on that "something else," because he has been brave enough to transform his approach to love-making.[77]

To help men be better lovers, he suggests they imagine what it's like to be a woman. He calls this "the journey of Tiresias."[78] Ferber invites the male reader to lie down on his back and relax, then takes him on a journey inside a woman's body. As he goes along, he is careful to reassure the man. He asks him to experience in his mind what a woman experiences in her body.

The journey begins with a very detailed description of the hidden regions of the woman's sexual organs: "the fragile, soft opening, edged with light, sensitive lips, [...] the wet warmth and the depth of the cave." Then the author asks the man to imagine the compelling desire to be penetrated, fulfilled, and filled, but not quickly or roughly. "No, feel the paradoxical need for a tender force that penetrates you very gently and slowly. Then feel your heart opening as the cave opens, welcomes and surrenders with delight to the back-and-forth movements of the penis inside it. Deep vibrations rise within you. Your body has lost its normal dimensions; it is dilated, enormous. Time and space no longer exist."[79]

Ferber realizes this is a difficult exercise, because it's asking men to be brave enough to identify with what a woman feels. But he also knows that when a man gets in touch with his feminine side he becomes much more in tune with a woman, and a better lover. He knows he doesn't have to be a phallic hero to satisfy a woman. He just needs to be present, between her legs, and if he can't penetrate her, place his penis at the entrance to what Taoists call "the precious door." The woman actually takes care of all the "penetrating" aspects of the man, including his voice, his loving words, his eyes, and his fingers—in other words, his presence.

"All the woman has to do is let him in and surrender. Everything happens inside her. She just has to open up, open up, open up ... And if the man is well and truly present, she will visit some very profound places on her own special journey."[80] Their two energies dance together, no longer knowing who is male and who is female, each absorbing the energy of the other, the yin of the woman and the yang of the man. You can stay like that, on the "plateau of pleasure," for a long time, basking in it and drawing energy from it. "And if an orgasm happens, ride the wave as if you are surfing."

The man feels the woman's orgasm as if it were his own. It's an overwhelming, mystical experience "to feel the tidal wave sweep over you and climb the ladder of your chakras, from the most primitive to the most spiritual, in an ethereal, glowing orgasm."[81] The orgasm described here is not explosive but implosive, spreading throughout the body.

Motionless union

IN ONE OF my earlier books,[82] I discussed the sexual relationship of an 80-year-old man and a 70-year-old woman who practiced "the Tao of love and sex,"[83] a Chinese spiritual way that advocates fully enjoying earthly and heavenly delights, including carrying on making love into old age, because making love feeds life.

It's important to understand that longevity is a highly esteemed value for the Chinese. As long as you remain healthy, old age is the happiest stage of life. A long and happy life depends on the coming together of the yin and yang energies of man and woman. I recall the old man telling me he virtually never had an erection anymore, but he still made love with his wife every day. They would hold each other, naked, and focus their attention on their genitals, enjoying the tender, thrilling feeling of their contact for many minutes, conscious that they were tapping into each other's energy to take what they needed to feel whole, in harmony, peaceful and happy to be alive. The pleasure he felt wasn't like a violent explosion, but a delicious relaxation. He had also learned how to separate orgasm from ejaculation, realizing that the latter (known as the *petite mort*—"little death"—in the West) is far less sensual than the feeling of cosmic union that holding back ejaculation can help you achieve. What the man experienced was a feeling of release, a voluptuous and sensual communion that extended into something bigger than himself.

The Tao of love and sex is a sensual practice that's perfectly suited to ageing couples, for many reasons. The Tao has no word for impotence, for example. The people of ancient China didn't consider it a major problem, because not having an erection doesn't stop an elderly man from creating the union of yin and yang. There are many ways of giving and receiving pleasure. If all ageing men wallowing in an "abyss of sadness," as Simone de Beauvoir wrote, were familiar with this approach to loving, they would realize that men can penetrate their partners without being erect.

In order to do so they need to know the "miraculous"[84] techniques of "soft penetration": the close contact of a penis and a vagina without erection. The couple must first learn to breathe slowly and deeply in order to relax. They must then open up, sharpen their senses, and not seek to achieve anything at all. The *Su Nu Ching*, a 19th-century erotic manual, states that one of the two may slowly move their pelvis from time to time to revitalize the union between the "jade stalk" and the "precious door" and so increase sensations.[85] This intimate exchange of energy creates a deep, nourishing connection. The manual recommends staying in that position for as long as you want, but at least a quarter of an hour, almost without moving.

"Not having an erection doesn't stop an elderly man from creating the union of yin and yang. There are many ways of giving and receiving pleasure."

You can make love like this, moving very little and very slowly, with fairly long pauses during which you simply feel the communion with your partner, observing your own pleasure. If an orgasm comes, so much the better, but it is not the goal. Not having a goal is profoundly liberating.

I remember the elderly couple telling me that on no account would they exchange the pleasure they experienced making love that way. "It is a delightful form of penetration," the wife said, reminding me that a woman's sexual satisfaction has very little to do with penis size. Su Nu, the teacher of Emperor Huang-Di, said the same thing: "If the man accompanies the union with his love and respect for the woman, and if he is deeply moved by what he's doing, what difference would a slight change in size or shape make? A hard member thrust roughly in and out is worth less than a soft member moving gently and delicately."[86]

Although the Taoists stress the importance of technique in love-making, it is the search for reciprocal harmony and serenity that matters most. The sexual act is not purely mechanical, but a total experience. Sensory development is fed by this harmonious sexuality: touch and smell, exchanging breath, prolonged bodily contact, gentle, slow caresses, and tenderly spoken words.

A Chinese doctor called Soen believed that once both partners have reached a high level of consciousness, "they become profoundly united while remaining motionless so as not to disturb the *king* (semen). They can practice this sort of union dozens of times in 24 hours. In so doing they will experience longevity."[87]

As I write this passage, I recall a story I was told a few years ago by a 60-year-old woman. It was about an affair she'd had 30 years earlier that had lasted six years, with a man who was much older than her and who she greatly admired for his talent as a speaker. One evening, after one of his lectures, she invited him back to her home, and they made love. He could no longer get an erection. Instead of being upset by it, the young woman sat on top of him with their genitals touching. They stayed like that, talking and whispering sweet nothings, in wonderful intimacy. To her surprise, she soon felt this very erotic contact between them creating the waves of an orgasm in her. One day she had one of the most intense orgasms she'd ever known. He, too, despite the apparent immobility of his penis, appeared to reach heights of ecstasy.

The woman is now 70 years old. She tells me that having sex with an impotent man doesn't worry her. She knows that it can be just as good, if not better, on condition that the man drop his guard, surrender, and abandon all images of his past sexuality. It can be an incredible adventure, she tells me. I realize, listening to her, that she has found true erotic freedom, and that she is a blessing for the man she makes love with.

The demands of a youth-obsessed culture

THESE EROTIC TECHNIQUES have been appropriated by Americans, who are fascinated by Eastern beliefs. Most of the books about slow sex are written in the United States and are devoured by baby boomers who want to stay young and sexually active.

The authors, all in their 60s, reveal that they have never felt as sexually fulfilled.[88] And this fact is confirmed by the United States of Aging Survey.[89] They are keen to share the keys to their success with their peers. Although they all convey the message that your sex life won't last post-60 without love, tenderness, and awareness, they struggle to shake off their generation's youth-obsessed demands.

I stumbled across a book published in the U.S. in 2006 about sex after 60.[90] The author, Joan Price, had put a classified ad in a newspaper: "Wanted: Interviews with sassy, sexy women, age 60+, who are willing to share feelings and experiences openly and anonymously in a candid, woman-to-woman book." Her book relates the positive sexual experiences of a selection of women (we aren't told how many contacted her) but leaves out any interviews she may have done with women who said they were relieved not to be having sex anymore.

Price begins by asking the question, "Why is it that making love after you're 60 is so good? Better than you'd ever expect?" Even though our organs are ageing and our

sensations are dulling? She recognizes that sexual fulfilment after 60 is less to do with the body, but more to do
with the head: "Sexual response is in our brains more than
our genitals."[91] What makes the difference is the fact that
women know themselves better, know their bodies better, know what gives them pleasure better, and know what
they want better. They are also wiser. If they are single,
they choose their partners better and look for mature men
with a spiritual side. They have a greater sense of intimacy,
especially if they no longer have the burden of children.

> "Sexual fulfilment after 60 is less to do with
> the body, but more to do with the head."

The author points out the difference between "physiological need" and "desire." She writes: "I'm having the
most wonderfully satisfying sex [...] I love and desire my
partner: the whole person he is [...] I love our intimacy."[92]
She says that when you are older, sexuality becomes
more "spiritual."

Up until that point I agree with her. She does a good job
of explaining that sexual fulfilment after 60 requires intimacy in the relationship. But the further into the book I
get, the more I wonder why she still falls into the trap of
a youth-obsessed culture—one that believes you must be
attractive and achieve orgasm at all costs to be sexually
fulfilled. The more I read, the more disappointed I am.
Women must be sexy, slim, have thighs of steel, and young
girl's legs—thanks to aerobics, hiking, and dancing—and

wrinkle-free faces. They must do their Kegel exercises every day to strengthen their pelvic-floor muscles and tone their perinea, and even carry a crystal stone egg in their vaginas as they do them. In short, they must *appear young*. That's the price they must pay to remain desirable, it seems. To be happy sexually, it is essential they achieve orgasm. And as it is harder for them to do so, because of their decreased libido and subdued sensations, they must use sex toys in order to be aroused. A whole section of the book resembles a catalogue of erotic objects and gadgets designed to help women climax.

Why this focus on performance, when the first part of the book tries to persuade us that sex is "so much better after 60" if you surrender to your partner and create a bond based on intimacy?

Orgasmic meditation

I WAS INTRODUCED to this rather unusual version of slow sex when a friend of mine gave me a book by Nicole Daedone that she'd brought back from the U.S.[93] Orgasmic meditation (OM) is a term coined by the lovely American author to describe a rather strange, albeit very structured and even timed practice that, according to Daedone, enables, "any man to bring out the orgasm in any woman in just 15 minutes."[94] The woman lies on her back, naked to the waist, legs spread apart, while the man caresses her clitoris very slowly and gently for 15 minutes. This technique involves shifting from "faster" and "stronger" to "slower" and "more connected." It isn't masturbation, she says; it's a form of meditation during which the person caressing and the person being caressed cast aside all expectations and fantasies so they are simply present, mindful of what is happening and of what each person is feeling. Expressing that sensation is part of the meditation and of the connection.

The numerous interviews published in the book all seem to confirm that OM leads to more intense, deeper orgasms, improves the quality of intimacy between the couple, brings about a sense of completeness, and gives them increasing desire to make love.

Even so, in the U.S., Orgasmic Meditation is considered a fringe activity practiced by an inner circle of experts. Although Daedone's philosophy is seen as "a refreshing counterpoint to pornography," it's hard to imagine the average American taking up this type of erotic meditation. It's even harder to imagine the average French senior citizen going on a group OM course, where there is no privacy at all, and trying to achieve an orgasm against the clock—the mere pressure of which takes away all the charm and romance of the activity.

• • •

CHAPTER EIGHT

Old-age love

Is ageing an obstacle to the joy of love? How does it evolve over a lifetime? And can desire last a lifetime?

• • •

"At the end of an unfamiliar corridor, a doorway caught my eye. Like a voyeur, I watched an elderly couple kissing. I felt like I had come across a pair of illicit lovers. There they were, a man and a woman, gently caressing each other's bodies. I couldn't hear what they were whispering to each other, but I could easily make out a few loving words, some of which sounded quite risqué. I had often wondered about sexuality in older people. And ultimately, it was a personal question: does desire die? [...] From that point on, my own love life has been continually informed by thoughts of old age. I've decided that you just have to let things happen and forget about boundaries, even forget about morality. Since then I've constantly felt the urgency of desire and constantly thought of sensuality as the essence of life. I believe we live differently when we live with this intimate awareness of old age."

David Foenkinos, *Les Souvenirs*[95]

Sexuality guided by the heart

IT'S HARD TO find the right tone to talk about sexuality in older people. The only way to do it is to show that it is *different*: internalized, infinitely gentler, slower, and more sensual. It is no longer guided by impulse, but by the heart. It is an emotional sexuality. The expression "to make love" has never been more meaningful than when used to describe the intimate, loving connection between two people who are ageing or already old. In his book *Pour une vieillesse ardente* ("For a Passionate Old Age"), the philosopher and psychoanalyst Roger Dadoun does not hesitate to call it erotic. And he's right, because *making love* is a way of being ageless. Lovers in the throes of passion are plunged into a timeless sensory experience, and nothing could be better for them.

We've read Macha Méril's account, and most of us have heard Jane Fonda's highly mediatized declarations: "At 74, I enjoy making love and I've never had such a fulfilling sex life." We've also read the reactions of "experts" who urge us not to "sell dreams" to older people, and who tell us to exercise caution, because—they say—ageing organs affect our ability to feel desire and experience pleasure.

"Making love is a way of being ageless."

So there are different points of view on the subject. I think the misunderstanding arises from what we mean by "a complete and satisfying sex life." A survey conducted among some 800 women in California over 40 years found that the oldest age group had the highest percentage of "sexual satisfaction."[96] While only 30 percent of sexually active women between 60 and 70 said they were "satisfied," almost half of octogenarians with an active sex life reported a "high level of orgasmic satisfaction." However, this research is contradicted by a Canadian study, which conversely found that, while advancing age has virtually no impact on the level of "sexual satisfaction" in men, it tends to decrease dramatically in women.[97]

I decided to take a closer look at the results of these studies. The Canadian study made a point of explaining that it was primarily interested in "coital activity," which tends to decrease with age. Older lovers prefer caresses and kisses, proving that there is more love than desire between them, and they hardly ever mention activities involving penetration. So the contradiction between the two studies comes from the different meaning given to the word "satisfying." In the American study, it refers not only to intercourse but to a group of intimate pleasures and gestures that are all the more powerful when they are part of a loving relationship and an "emotional and physical closeness with a partner."

You won't understand a thing about shared eroticism in older people if you don't value intimacy. And what is intimacy, if not the ability to reveal who you are to your partner and accept them as they are? What is intimacy, if not the mutual acceptance of one another's vulnerability? This involves trust and tenderness. The quest for sexual love among older people is challenging, because this sought-after intimacy brings couples out of their "narcissistic shell." According to Yann Dall'Aglio in his book *Jt'm, l'amour est-il has been?* ("Is Love Has-been?"), it has less to do with "common tastes or interests, but with an avowed weakness for each other that is part and parcel of the human condition."[98] He asks what is genuine intimacy, if not the desire to witness one's beloved age? What truly loving rapport does not include the shared fatigue, awkwardness, and "the gradual, distressing withering of both partners?"[99]

Since baby boomers have been raised on the concepts of self-control and performance, they have no other choice as they grow older and approach death but to carry out their narcissistic revolution. They are compelled to do so. One 72-year-old man, whose wife had died four years earlier, and who had just met a woman his age, told me, "The woman I hold in my arms and lovingly caress is no 'sex bomb.' Her body is old and vulnerable yet tender, and vibrates with emotions. I find it touching. And when my body moves towards hers and hers towards mine, it's like we're dancing. Every embrace, gentle or strong, is a union."

This is why there is so much tenderness and humor in the love ageing couples lavish on each other.

They must still make love

I FINISH READING *La joie d'amour* ("The Joy of Love") by Robert Misrahi[100] while on a ferry returning from the Île d'Yeu, a beautiful island off the coast of the Loire region in France. The boat is crammed with holidaymakers, mostly families from the wealthy Paris suburb of Versailles with young children, all tanned and full of energy. The parents, successful 40- and 50-somethings, are active, fast, do five things at once, talk quickly and loudly, and take up all the room—including that of a discreet, elegant older couple that is vainly trying to preserve its own personal space.

I observe this couple and am suddenly struck by the startling contrast between their peaceful faces and the whirlwind of indifferent younger people around them. They are both beautiful—the kind of beauty that emanates from within. Eyes closed and leaning on each other tenderly, they seem to be experiencing a happiness that is beyond reach for the others. The man has a soft, mysterious smile as he strokes his wife's hand slowly and sensually. They are in a world of their own, far removed from the surrounding chaos, and as I watch them I'm surprised to feel an unexpected sense of calm and joy wash over me. The sight of them makes me feel good, and I realize that I'm the only person who can tell what they're experiencing, silently and unbeknownst to everyone else.

They must still make love, I tell myself—I'm sure of it! They wouldn't be so connected, so serene and happy together, if they weren't physically intimate. Of course, I'll never be able to prove it, but I've learned to tell whether an older couple has a lasting physical relationship by the aura they give off.

Misrahi asks if ageing—the slow advance of old age—is an obstacle to the joy of love. Not if you enjoy the kind of loving closeness I've just been speaking of; not if you are connected, tender, caring, and affectionate with each other. Can you be totally in harmony with someone in both body and spirit?

Octogenarians who want to make love

I WATCH THE couple on the ferry throughout lunch. He is very elegant and well-dressed, but also elderly and quite frail. She is much more lively, even though she seems roughly the same age as he is. She's still beautiful, with regular features, blue eyes, and a slender figure. They sit beside each other. He looks at her lovingly, and she keeps putting her hand on his affectionately.

It's so rare to see this kind of public display of affection between a couple of 80-somethings that I simply have to go over and introduce myself. I tell them about my book on the future of loving intimacy, and ask if they would mind being included. I obviously have no idea what's really going on between them, but their overt display of love intrigues me. She seems very open to my proposal from the outset: "We met each other again two years ago, after a 40-year gap. Pierre had just lost his wife and was single. We are in love." Although I'm dying to know more, and she seems ready to pour her heart out, I tell them I'd prefer to visit them in their home in Burgundy.

A few weeks later, I go for lunch at their house—or rather at his, because I find out that they don't live together yet. She's Italian and lives in Rome, but is renting a small studio apartment in the neighboring town to his, Joigny, so she can visit him every so often. He also goes to Rome to stay with her. When I arrive, he's got a bad case of bronchitis and greets me in a very elegant dressing gown. I've already noticed his impeccable sense of style, which shows he cares about his appearance and respects others. He kisses my hand gently, which also impresses me. Then he apologizes for not being able to join us for lunch. She—Marisa—will take me out for lunch to a good restaurant in town, and we'll return for coffee with him afterwards.

I then realize he probably wants his partner to speak with me first. Perhaps he's a bit uncomfortable about the interview? When you're 80, talking about sex with a writer who clearly intends to publish your account is never going to be easy. But I later find out that he devoured my book on ageing, which I sent them in preparation for our meeting.[101] The pages have been annotated, particularly the ones about sexuality in the chapter called "A Sensual Old Age." This reassures me, and I then think we'll be able to discuss the subject quite easily.

Marisa and I are in the restaurant. I'm struck by how confidently she tells me their story. They first met 40 years ago in Italy, but he was married, so nothing came of it. Marisa, on the other hand, never married. Rich and beautiful, she's led the life of an independent, highly cultured woman with a passion for psychology and spirituality. She's had many lovers over the years. Looking at her, I imagine she must have been one of those irresistibly attractive modern Italian women who paid dearly for her freedom in a male chauvinist world. The price she paid was solitude. She realized it rather late in life but was able to express it. So when a friend of hers heard that Pierre had been widowed, she arranged for them to meet again.

"I wanted a partner," she admits. He'd been through some hard times, first his cancer, which he recovered from, then his wife's, which she died from. Like many men, he hated the idea of living alone, so he pursued Marisa eagerly. "He wrote a really moving letter asking me if I'd agree to take the place of his wife." Marisa had no intention of replacing his wife, or of becoming his nurse, so they negotiated a lifestyle that allowed them to keep some of their independence.

"He's more in love with me than I am with him," she tells me, but he had "such a lovely way of kissing me on the mouth that he won my heart. We love each other, and we are octogenarians who want to make love." She corrects herself: "I want to make love with him, but it's complicated. It's been so long since he had sex. We're seeing a sex therapist who's trying to help us." I realize that she still has quite a youthful libido and dreams of having a full sexual relationship. But he, like many men his age, hasn't had an erection for quite some time and basically doesn't have much of a libido anymore. But he loves her, wants to satisfy her, and is prepared to put a lot of effort into doing so—which includes discussing their problem with a young, 45-year-old sex therapist. I must admit I think they're both very brave.

Marisa: "We love each other, and we are octogenarians who want to make love."

An hour later, I have coffee with Pierre, who is feeling a little better. He tells me that this young sex expert has tried to explain that an 80-year-old's sexuality is quite different from a 40-year-old's. Instead of focusing on performance, they must explore each other's bodies and be affectionate with each other.

"We don't have time to make love," he tells me. I can't help laughing. Don't have time? Marisa tells me they don't have a bed! Or rather, a double bed. They sleep in twin beds, so they never get to curl up with each other and cuddle. In the evenings, after dinner, they both fall straight to sleep. During the few sessions they had with their sex therapist, they realized that they urgently needed to buy themselves a double bed. That bed will be arriving shortly. Then they will be able to take an afternoon nap together and "make affection"—a different way of making love.

Hearing them talk so directly about their intimate life together is both surprising and moving. "In your book," exclaims Pierre, "you say that a woman can experience fulfilment through genital contact, even if the man doesn't have an erection. But Marisa expects me to have one! Otherwise she gets frustrated. I'm wondering whether I should take Viagra." Why not, I reply, recalling that François Parpaix told me he'd prescribed Viagra to a 96-year-old, because he needed to feel like a man again.

I then consider how deeply ingrained these symbols of virility are for men and women alike. They threaten the development of physical intimacy in old age. How many men would rather give up their sex lives than explore another way of making love? And how many older women also remain obsessed with the memory of their youthful experiences, convinced that the only way to achieve sexual pleasure is to be penetrated? I feel that Pierre and Marisa's relationship has reached a turning point. If they want to experience their love fully, and experience it with their bodies and souls, they must abandon their reference points and open their minds to something new: snuggle up to each other in the double bed that's about to arrive and let things happen.

They are also intelligent enough to understand the danger of wanting to reproduce what they've experienced in the past. It's bound to end in failure.

"Making affection"–a different way of making love

I FIRST HEARD that lovely expression from an older couple who still made love, but in a different way. André (89) and Jeanne (85) have lived with each other for 65 years. They are in fairly good health and independent. It's obvious they are happy together, and very close. I sense it from the outset in the way they behave, both individually, in their calm, glowing demeanor, and with each other, since they gently radiate positive energy that unites them like a kind of invisible halo. You feel good around them, which is significant. They exude happiness.

We talk about their relationship. I learn that they "got married for life" and that despite the challenges and hard times, their marriage has lasted because they have always been faithful to each other and trusted each other implicitly. André tells me, "I've always thought that when you're faced with temptation—and I have been—there can't be a first time. When a man cheats on his wife once, he opens a door that will never be closed again!" Jeanne adds, "I've always trusted him. I've always known that I could lean on him if I had a problem." The affectionate closeness that emanates from them now, in their old age, is based on physical closeness, an attraction they've always had for each other.

I look at them and think they are both beautiful. André has an elegance about him, a poised masculinity, and handsome eyes that convey integrity and self-confidence and make you want to reach out to him. Jeanne has a pretty, feminine face that exudes a soft, understated sensuality, but also a certain strength. I ask them a rather intimate question: how has their sexuality evolved over the past 65 years? They are both more than happy to answer me. She instantly replies that it has constantly gotten better over time. Of course, after the honeymoon period of the first three years, there were times when she felt less interested, because she was pregnant or busy with the children, and he also had moments when he was worn down by work and stress. But over the years, they've continued to enjoy making love. "We *did it* for a very long time." I realize that they probably don't *do it* anymore, but I don't want to ask them when they stopped *doing it*, because I get the impression that they've found another way of being sensual and affectionate with each other.

Jeanne makes a point of telling me that they've never had separate rooms and have always slept in the same bed. They even cuddle each other and hold hands before falling asleep, and she says that this loving contact between their bodies and skin has been vital for her. Then she talks about their dancing. They have always loved to dance, first ballroom and then country. At this point, André gets excited. He tells me about the time they were on a skiing trip with a group of older people and they took part in a dance evening at their hotel, which was full of young executives. They started dancing waltzes, tangos, and paso dobles, and the young people came over to congratulate them, saying how

much they enjoyed watching them and what a rare pleasure it was to see their old bodies moving so beautifully in
time with the music. They were good dancers, and it was
obvious they were enjoying it. The young people couldn't
get over it! They had the proof right before their eyes that
you could still dance and make love late in life.

Ultimately, André and Jeanne cultivate the pleasure
of an understanding rapport just like you cultivate a garden, with care and awareness. Pleasure is central to their
relationship, even when they share their problems. They
pay attention to each other, talk a lot, and never "have a
go at each other." They know how lucky they are to still be
together, and they thank God—who they believe in—every
day for this good grace.

"Yes, we're lucky, because a lot of our friends of our age
tolerate each other but don't love each other anymore. They
fill a mutual vacuum, but they're not happy." They both
consider their good luck to be a fragile and precarious gift,
because although they no longer worry about "temptations"
rocking their relationship, they know that death awaits
them and that they will have to leave each other one day. So
their relationship is not a safety net, a rampart, or a guaran-
tee against solitude. It doesn't protect them at all. It's a risk.

They certainly are lucky to still be together at their age.
I think of all the men and women who would love to experience such a serene, affectionate closeness but who find
themselves alone, widowed or divorced, and who have
already crossed love off their list of future plans. Solitude has made those people calmly pessimistic. They seem
to have grown used to the loss of their love life and sex
life, but often at the cost of a kind of sad resignation that

makes them grow older rapidly. I also think of all the couples who haven't made love for a long time but who stay together for all sorts of valid reasons, from habit to the fear of being alone. Sometimes I catch their eye in the Parisian restaurants I dine in. They don't say a word to each other throughout their meal, concentrate on eating their food, at most mutter some comment about the wine or dish, but don't talk to each other, and look bored. They are definitely not going to make love when they get home. Their solitary pastimes await them—surfing the internet, reading, and watching TV. Eros left a long time ago.

Desire can last a lifetime

DR OLIVIER SOULIER has a few stories to share when I talk to him about my interest in old-age love. The first patient he tells me about is a 90-year-old widow. He describes her as extremely charming, very coquettish, and still very attractive. What does he put this down to? Probably the fact that she has always had sexual desires and still does. "My secret to longevity is pleasure," she once told him. Gabrielle spent her entire life with the same man, on a wine estate in the Languedoc. She met her husband when she was 20 years old and never went with another man. Desire was central to their relationship, and at 80 years old and counting she said they still made love two or three times a week. If Robert was busy in his office and she felt like having sex, she wouldn't think twice about flirting with him until he made love to her. One day Robert had a fatal accident. Gabrielle manifested her grief through various psychosomatic symptoms, including bouts of cystitis and vaginal itching.

She came to Olivier for a consultation, and since he's known her well for a long time, he spoke frankly with her: "Do you miss Robert? Do you still want to make love with him?" Gabrielle broke down: "How can anyone understand that an 85-year-old woman still wants to make love, Doctor?" Olivier asked her if she touched herself from time to time. Gabrielle exclaimed in surprise—no, never. Her man always took good enough care of her in that respect.

Gabrielle: "My secret to longevity is pleasure."

A few months later, she returned for another consultation. Her vaginal itching had disappeared. Gabrielle then admitted that she'd thought a lot about what her doctor had suggested. So she touched herself, and, to her astonishment, she felt Robert was there with her. It was as if he was touching her himself. Olivier told me he wasn't the least bit surprised. Your skin and body have a memory. When your entire erotic life is imprinted on your body, you'll find it again. Gabrielle now knows how to maintain her connection with Robert and their whole love story, and she has rekindled the flame of her desire, which keeps her healthy at her ripe old age.

Olivier, who has seen many people in his consulting room over the years, is convinced that a couple's love life and sex life can last a lifetime, "as long as their relationship is strong enough to fan the flame of desire, however small." He remembers staying with an elderly couple as a young medic. In the mornings, as he was drinking his coffee half asleep, he'd see the man approach his wife by the stove, push her against it, and rub himself against her with delight. They would both laugh. They actually slept in separate rooms, because he disturbed her with his snoring. Olivier thought, as any 25-year-old would, that they no longer had a sex life. But he saw this was not the case: they told him quite matter-of-factly that they always made time "for a cuddle" in the evening or morning. They had a funny code. He would come into the bedroom and say, "Madame, nature calls," to which she would laugh and reply, "May God's will be done!" A few years later, Olivier found out that they had both died within three months of each other. Couples like this who are intensely bonded and sexually attracted to each other often die close together. The survivor soon follows the one who goes first.

"When your entire erotic life is imprinted
on your body, you'll find it again."

These old-age loves only stay together because of the high quality of their relationship, concludes Olivier. Some men in their 80s can still get enough of an erection to penetrate their wives, even if it doesn't last as long or happen as often. It's because they feel loved and desired. But it's not just about the man's sex drive. The woman's attitude is just as important. "The woman can sometimes make or break the man," says Olivier. To illustrate his point, he tells me about a 60-year-old businessman whose "difficult" wife humiliated him non-stop by telling him he was a bad lover, until he ended up leaving her. When he was 70 he met a woman of 65. Since he hadn't made love for ten years, he'd completely lost his "erectile function." His new partner didn't think it was important. They invented their own erotic game and gave each other pleasure in a different way. Two years later, his erection came back.

This demonstrates, says Olivier, that a man who can "no longer get a hard-on" can still regain his virility with a gentle, loving partner. "You just need time and love."

Erotic relationships beyond the grave

CERTAIN EROTIC RELATIONSHIPS are so strong that they even continue after death. It's a taboo subject that few people are willing to discuss, but some widowers and widows have dared to open up about it. I spoke about this with the author Noëlle Châtelet, who was brave enough to broach the subject in one of her novels, *Madame George*.[102] The protagonist, Mme Mansour, is a 75-year-old widow who is devastated after the loss of her husband. With her long plait, more white than blonde, arranged sensibly on her chest, hunched up with sadness, she tells her psychiatrist about the presence of her husband, who is dead. She evokes all the grief of a woman who suddenly finds herself without her man. Without *him*.

"As I told you the other day, doctor, my husband has started joining me at night. I've always made sure I leave enough room for him on the right-hand side of our bed, his side. I would never dare sleep on that side. I've never moved over from my side. I really don't need that much room. When he comes to me, it's very sweet, very comforting. He doesn't come every night. But I wake up when he does. I know when he's there. It's hard to say ... Usually, I can tell by the change in temperature. It suddenly feels warmer, or colder, above my head. The air quivers, sometimes so precisely that it feels like he's stroking my hair. He really loved my hair, and never wanted me to cut it, you see. Then the mattress sinks, but so softly, so imperceptibly that I can barely feel it ... yet there's definitely an extra weight on the bed. Not like before ... Before his death."

The psychiatrist asks her if it's a weightless weight. "Yes, that's it, doctor. Exactly. And I can sense a shape, too, if I turn my head to his side of the bed, in the darkness. It's hard to explain ..." The psychiatrist continues: "Do you mean a shapeless shape, invisible yet defined, looking at you not with eyes, but with eyes that have become an idea, an abstract idea ... The idea of eyes, is that it, Madame Mansour?"[103]

The lovely 70-something is not afraid of what is happening to her, of the presence of her husband in her bed. "I'm so happy to be reunited with him like this! It proves that he's thinking of me, like I think of him! In the end, there's no clean break between the dead and the living. There are pathways. I'm convinced of it."[104]

Noëlle Châtelet has said that she has personally experienced what she describes in her novel. Many others have also felt the physical presence of someone they've loved. At a recent conference, I heard Noëlle ask whether these "intangible bodies" are created by the sensory imagination, or whether science would eventually be able to prove that they are real.[105]

Wisdom is knowing when to stop

IN LUDOVIC VIROT'S 2011 documentary film *Le sens de l'âge* ("The Meaning of Ageing"), several octogenarians speak candidly about how their sex drive and love life have changed.

Sitting on a bench in winter, an old man of 80 tells us: "I feel just as capable of loving now as I did 20 or 40 years ago. Just as capable. But I still need to find the right window of opportunity and the right partner. The last time I felt a sexual urge was fairly recently, 4 years ago. I became quite infatuated with someone, as I always do. But nothing came of it. Now I lead a quiet life and don't lust after anybody, but I'm not frustrated at all. I'll wait for my sex drive to reappear—maybe it will and maybe it won't! I think it's possible to have a full loving relationship at any age. In any case, the *hope* of love remains alive, however old you are."

Next we meet Madeleine, also 80, who lives alone in Paris's Chinatown and has made friends with a group of young people. They take her to the market on their scooters, invite her out for drinks, and they've even taught her to play table tennis and introduced her to manicures. In short, she seems to be having a good time with them. When Virot asks what life is like for her now, she admits to missing her husband's affection: "You never forget the physical contact you had with a husband you loved. I don't see myself starting over with another man. Anyway, I'm too old. I don't have the same desires or needs as I had at 60." It's been ten years since she had a "man in the house," and she says she doesn't even think about it. "But I must admit that I do notice good-looking men, attractive ones—and beautiful women, for that matter! I'll say to my girlfriend, 'Look how handsome he is.'"

But it stops there. Would she like to have physical contact with an attractive man?

"Oh, no!" she exclaims. "It wouldn't cross my mind. I envy women who can still do that. I don't see myself meeting anyone now and having a romantic relationship. No—I couldn't even think about it! I'm not saying I wouldn't meet up with someone to go to an exhibition. But I never want another bloke around the house. I've had enough of that, and I'm not doing it again," she laughs, adding: "I'm happy spending time with my girlfriends!"

We then see Robert, 90, in his bathroom, where he's practicing Tai Chi, sound therapy, and advanced stretching techniques. His energy is impressive, and he works hard at it. He says he's very happy now, after a life that's had its ups and downs, and he enjoys "his independence." When asked about falling in love at his age, he laughs. "Being in love is like being sick. You don't see clearly. You don't see the real person. You're blind! I've been in love and it's crazy, you lose all your common sense, all your logic!" No—being in love now is out of the question.

Frida, 85, doesn't see herself falling in love either. She lives in a beautiful property where she hosts seminars. She also seems very happy with her life, surrounded by her plants, which she tends to lovingly, and her guests, who she bakes delicious cakes for and plays board games with. When Virot asks her about her sexual desires, she's very forthright: "Let's get things straight. I'm not looking. My granddaughter tried to convince me that it would be good for me to have someone. I replied that I'd like to find a pal, a friend, but a platonic one—someone who could take me to the cinema, drive my car, whisk me away on holiday. 'At my age, what more can I hope for?' I told her."

Madeleine: "I envy women who can still do that. I don't see myself meeting anyone now and having a romantic relationship. No—I couldn't even think about it!"

Frida says that all her close friends are dead, and that after a certain age you don't make really good friends anymore like you did when you were 20. "There's a very kind gentleman who comes to help me with my bees. He's 90 years old. I'm 85, so it's a respectable age gap! Poor thing, though. He's always tired, even though he still drives his car and looks after his bees. But I can't live with someone who's got no energy and who wants to go to bed early, when I don't feel like going to bed early. Even if we don't share the same room, if I want to play cards one evening and he's sleepy, it's not worth living together. So it gets difficult after a certain age. It's different for people who've lived together their whole lives. They know each other's faults, perhaps only too well. It might be unbearable for them, but it's not the end of the world. No—you can't start a new relationship when you're too old." Asked if she might fall in love one day, she grins, but is categorical: "No, I don't think so." Why not? "First of all, because the men in my life have given me everything I could have asked for from a man—brains, good looks, and love. I've had all that, and don't need a replacement, because whoever I found now would only be a pale imitation of who I had before. It's not worth it. And I don't feel like it anyway. I'm perfectly fine as I am."

Frida then brings up all the gratuitous sex scenes in films. "I just think: here we go, more gymnastics! It's different when you're young. You have sexual desires. At my age you don't feel desire anymore. Wisdom is knowing when to stop. Anyway," she adds with a bright smile, "it stops on its own. And it's no loss. You just change. You become different."

Looking kindly on sexuality in old people

I OFTEN HEAR that the younger generation finds the idea of sexuality in old people unimaginable. Sometimes the words are even harsher: "disgusting," even "perverse." So you'll understand why I was so surprised to meet a young film-maker of 38 who looks kindly on old-age sexuality.

We meet for coffee at Café de Flore in Paris. Andrea Riedinger talks passionately about the news stories she has shot in the United States, particularly the one on "merry widows." She remembers Naomi Wilzig, the woman who founded the World Erotic Art Museum in Miami, the largest erotic-art collection in the world. By the time she died, in 2015, aged 80, she had amassed more than 4,000 erotic works of art, dating from 300 BCE to the present day, including paintings, sculptures, sex toys, and other objects. She built her unique collection with the colossal inheritance she received after the death of her billionaire banker husband, who did not approve of her interest in erotic art. Before she died she lived in an apartment overlooking the sea with her partner, a black man called Jessie who was half her age. She was completely comfortable with her sexuality till the very end and became a sort of sex therapist and counsellor to younger women.

Andrea also tells me about Dolores, who, having been widowed at 80, is "following her dreams" and has even competed in the Miss Arkansas Senior beauty pageant. Andrea filmed her going to meet her younger lover at the airport. "You should have seen how gorgeous they looked!" she says. "There was so much love in her eyes, and their reunion was so wonderful, that I wanted to be in their shoes!"

This is the first time I've heard a young woman speak kindly, even a little enviously, about the sexuality of a woman old enough to be her grandmother. It's nice to hear!

In retirement homes

SEXUALITY IN ELDERLY people will probably remain taboo for a long time, perhaps forever, for reasons that are more subconscious than cultural. In the same way that children can't imagine their parents making love, young people can't conceive of older adults as sexual beings. It's probably why sexuality is so looked down upon in retirement homes.

However, the right to privacy and therefore to intimacy is one of our basic human rights, as ministers responsible for the elderly keep reminding us year after year. Not respecting the sexuality of older people is quite simply a form of abuse. Our attitudes have certainly changed, but some caregivers still feel very uncomfortable, even embarrassed, by older people's sexual behavior, especially when they openly engage in that behavior in front of them.

"If the pleasure of love in our final years were limited to being together, showing affection, pecks on the cheek, and the warmth of physical contact, everyone would be fine with it, and in retirement homes we wouldn't hesitate to celebrate the fact that growing older can still mean having pleasure. All would be well, in an ideal world; the problem is that even in our final years, the pleasure of love is not always strictly limited to affection."[106]

"Not respecting the sexuality of older people is quite simply a form of abuse."

And in those cases, this "pleasure of love" is harshly condemned as ugly, dirty, and inappropriate. Caregivers will then ask doctors for drugs to control residents' sexual urges. Or their children will ask the staff to separate the "suitors." Arguments citing dementia, presumed lack of consent, or the safety of dependents in care often explains the intolerance of families and retirement home staff towards this sexual behavior.[107] But all these "good reasons" for depriving elderly people of their intimacy and sexuality are rooted in the difficulty we have collectively in imagining erotic desire in older adults and accepting that we may continue to need physical closeness, affection, and pleasure throughout our lives.

These issues are increasingly being addressed in training programs designed for retirement-home staff. Once caregivers are made aware of residents' continuing need for intimacy, they are able to respect it. "It's about helping professionals understand that sexuality and feelings are ageless," says Éric Seguin, the young director of a group of retirement homes in Finistère, Brittany (north-west France), "and thinking of residents' rooms as their homes, enabling the elderly person to have a space where they can be alone," he continues. "It also means taking the risk that you can't control everything and allowing the secret life of the institution to continue behind closed doors and with the lights out ..."[108] Seguin also believes that retirement-home rooms should be equipped with double beds, "because single beds are too cramped for lovemaking."

Ten years ago Paulette Guinchard (the French minister responsible for the elderly at the time) pointed out that state-assisted living accommodation only offered single beds, clearly showing that sexuality was "officially denied, if not prohibited."

When I started writing this book I heard about a French website called Quinquessence.fr that specializes in "Eroticism, culture and sexuality after 50" and also sells erotic items.[109] On Valentine's Day the site launched an awareness campaign called "Please respect my privacy" to encourage retirement-home staff to respect the intimacy of their residents. The statement on the company website read: "This special occasion is an opportunity to remind you that older people in assisted-living accommodation sometimes find it difficult to express their loving feelings without being patronized or disapproved of by members of staff. We are therefore helping facilities that have committed to setting up procedures to respect their residents' privacy by providing them with signs that read 'Please respect my privacy. Do not disturb,' which residents may hang on their bedroom doors."

To what extent should privacy be respected?

TODAY I AM having lunch with Annie de Vivie, a woman I've long admired for her commitment to improving care for older people. Annie runs Agevillage.com, a website dedicated to the support and care of elderly people, and works tirelessly to promote the concept of "humanitude" in retirement homes.[110] In the course of our conversation we discuss the need to strengthen the self-esteem of older people to prevent loss of independence, and I mention my own research. She then tells me the following story, which was also the subject of a presentation during her most recent seminar on Alzheimer's disease.

An elderly lady of 99 was regularly harming herself by masturbating with various inappropriate objects, in particular, her hairbrush. She was hospitalized several times for vulval and vaginal bleeding, after which the director of the care home met with her staff and decided to buy a sex toy for the resident. To leave things as they were would have meant not assisting someone in danger. They had to do something. And it was out of the question to deprive this elderly lady of objects she could use to satisfy a compelling need to give herself pleasure, a need that was perfectly natural and respectable.

"As you can imagine, it wasn't easy to persuade all the staff to agree to buy a dildo for a resident," Annie tells me. But the staff had been trained in the "humanitude" philosophy, and the idea of respecting the intimacy of elderly people, however vulnerable, was already firmly established in the care home. They informed the old lady's guardian, who was very open to the suggestion and understood the importance of this course of action. The director then bought the object and brought it to the old lady, who exclaimed, "Willy!" and immediately hid it in a box of chocolates. She was never rushed to hospital again for bleeding. The care-home staff said that one day, the resident's nephew opened the chocolate box and became very angry. How did a sex toy end up in his aunt's box of confectionary? The staff had to explain their whole decision-making process to the gentleman, who was very shocked by the discovery. They no doubt also had to broach the subject of old-age sexuality with the man—as well as, in this instance, the need to respect his aunt's privacy.

Agevillage.com reported that the elderly lady jokingly said she would have preferred a handsome young man, but "Willy kept her company till the end of her days."

CONCLUSION

• • •

WHAT HAVE I learned from this journey to the land where the older generation lives out their desires and loves—a land that is quite isolated, relatively unexplored, and fairly mysterious?

The sex experts I spoke to warned me not to be naive. And not to let ageing people think they would discover some exotic paradise.

After explaining in great detail how sexual ageing adversely affects our bodies, they also acknowledged that we can continue to feel love and desire as we grow older and experience wonderful new things—namely, a different kind of Eros (sexual love). But that kind of erotic intimacy involves putting the familiar behind us, surrendering to what we feel, and not worrying about our image.

In other words, a true narcissistic revolution is required. We must stop looking in the mirror. We must stop seeking reassurance from our partner and build a bond based on intimacy with them instead, which includes physical pleasure.

According to the men and women who are experiencing this slower, more sensual sexuality with the person they love, age doesn't take away any of the joy from love. Quite the opposite. It even lets you combine sex and tenderness, something that can be hard when you're young and caught in the throes of passion.

"We must stop looking in the mirror. We must stop seeking reassurance from our partner and build a bond based on intimacy with them instead, which includes physical pleasure."

The first condition is to keep feeling desire and love, whether you are alone or in a relationship. In other words, to keep living. To love life and being alive, and to stay open to new experiences.

The second condition is to have self-esteem, which involves taking care of yourself, your body, and your mind in order to remain desirable.

The third condition is to keep a certain distance from your loved one, in order to keep the mystery alive, while at the same time creating intimacy in everyday life. You create and maintain intimacy through distance and closeness. Without intimacy there can neither be Eros nor long-lasting love.

These conditions exclude older people who suffer from depression, bitterness, or despair, those who let themselves go, and those who have decided to draw a line through their sex lives for various reasons.

There are those who have never liked having sex or are too inhibited and those who are shackled by social or religious taboos, who feel guilty practicing their sexuality at an age when they have been freed from the duty to procreate, and who are victims of what Nietzsche referred to as the return of "Moralin" (that is, hypocritical, prudish morality).[111] I want to remind all those people that Pope John Paul II, who was more of a personalist than a theologian, tried (albeit rather unsuccessfully) to promote sexual pleasure as something good. Since people not only *have* a body but *are* a body, "flesh is no longer a 'mistake' or a 'curse.' It is part of people, and people are truly made to give themselves to each other. By giving themselves, they find themselves, and in so doing they find their happiness."[112] In the same book, Yves Semen quotes John Paul II as saying, "Pleasure is good because it is the very 'sign' of the full communion of two people who give themselves to each other through the intimacy of their bodies."

Some of the men and women who have drawn a line through their sex lives have done so because sex just doesn't interest them anymore. The phenomenon of asexuality intrigues me. I see a link between the consumerism of sex, the promotion of orgasms as compulsory, and the absence of desire, which some people declare as a status in its own right and as a release.

Others have given up on the pleasure of love because they're on their own. Women especially fall into this category, and loneliness is a real problem. I realized this after meeting many women who have agreed to conduct secret affairs because their lovers aren't free, or who go looking for soulmates on dating sites. I view the latter as a rather adolescent, idealistic activity, though I do know couples who have got together that way and are very happy. Meeting these people has shown me that it's a natural human instinct to continue to feel desire and to crave love and physical contact, regardless of age. But what has really surprised me is how creative they are in their pursuit of those things. The women learn what love really is—an act of surrendering to and trusting their partner, who they must accept for who they are and where they've come from. I've been touched by the men and women who have told me how their experiences in older age have made them change the way they love, for example, by being less possessive and more in tune with their partner. Most of them are able to live in the present and enjoy it without looking ahead to the future. They have reached an age when the present counts the most, because they have nothing left to build or improve, apart from the quality of their relationship.

I have taken an interest in how couples stand the test of time and continue to experience gentle, loving connectedness. Some people, who have had enough of sex, don't make love anymore; they "make affection." They still experience the joy of love and physical contact. They enjoy the softness of each other's skin, their smell, their warmth, and the sound of their voice. All these things feed love. This enduring need for physical contact proves that it is key to enjoying life.

Other older people learn new erotic practices, such as those developed in India and China over millennia. Together they explore another way of making love—one that's slower, more aware, and infinitely better suited to their ageing bodies than the impulsive sex they had when they were young. I ventured off to explore the Tantric way myself, on a course that taught me a lot. Now I understand better why so many youthful older people are interested in *this different sexuality*, whose goal is not to achieve orgasm but to become more connected with their partner through erotic communion. A more spiritual sexuality, you could say, since what they seek is an intimate connection on a deeper level—with the other person's mind, body, and soul.

"The enduring need for physical contact
proves that it is key to enjoying life."

As we age, the quality of our orgasms changes. They become more expansive, intense, and satisfying. They no longer have that dark, impulsive, almost involuntary side that carries your whole being like a violent wave, an experience that's more instinctive than *aware*. When we grow old, our bodies are no longer "desiring-machines," to quote French philosopher Gilles Deleuze. Just as well! Our bodies become sensitive bodies experienced from within, *animate corporalities*.

This is why Robert Misrahi ventures to say that when physical rapture is experienced *with awareness*, it gains in richness and significance. "When the loved person perceives him- or herself, through their partner, as exquisite skin and flesh, they do not feel objectified (as people sometimes believe). On the contrary, their very being is affirmed by this incarnation: they are the body-subject that is loved and admired. [...] Touch then becomes the joint gateway to a sweet ecstasy [...] so each person recognizes the presence of love in their own excitement. [...] In the joy and pleasure of love, each person delights in the existence of their partner as both flesh and spirit, each person offers the other and receives from the other a sort of *total presence*."[113]

Misrahi also paraphrases the following statement by the poet Paul Valéry: "The most profound thing about man is his skin." When we have skin-to-skin contact with another person, we discover what is unfamiliar and unique about them.

For many, an important aspect of growing old is exploring the happiness that can be derived from erotic physical contact. Physical pleasure doesn't just mean erotic and genital excitement. "Active joy" fills our bodies and minds: "Shared joy, through which the lovers are carried off together towards extreme rapture."[114]

I ended my journey in the land of old-age love. It exists everywhere but is often hidden because society doesn't look on it kindly or compassionately. Having said that, we are becoming increasingly aware of the abuse we inflict on the elderly by not respecting their privacy.

I hope I've helped to change people's opinions about what the future holds for us and about our freedom to love and desire as we grow older. By protecting that freedom into old age, we can hope to achieve a fulfilled life. Throughout this book I've attempted to show that the changes our bodies undergo as we age do not prevent us from having access to "higher sexual pleasure."[115] We can achieve it through awareness, surrendering to our partner, and, lastly, intimacy. It is a path to fulfilment, because when we've experienced "the irrefutable presence of love" in our lives, the joy of fulfilment naturally ensues.

AFTERWORD

• • •

WHEN *SEX AFTER SIXTY* was first published in France, I received so many reader responses that I decided to write an afterword for future editions, published under a different title: *Age, Desire, and Love*. I had initially envisioned that only my fellow sexagenarians would want to read the book, but I discovered that wasn't the case, that younger generations were also interested. I also never imagined that my forays into Tantra would spur so many questions, especially from women. Lastly, I presumed the book was mainly geared towards senior citizens in good health, but I came to realize that the frail also related to the material and would have liked to hear more about eroticism for the more fragile elderly.

The first surprise resulted from the interest shown by younger journalists regarding my book. Following an interview, one of them even confided in me that as she was about to turn 50, she too was fascinated by the subject matter, as older age was just around the corner. A radio-show host was also clearly touched by my views on the role that women can play as initiators in pursuing a happy sex life in older age. I also learned that he then heartily promoted my work at a conference organized by an insurance company. Yet the reaction of a 25-year-old Belgian journalist is what shocked me the most. She confessed that she was recommending this inventive book about sexuality to all her friends. Even my 22-year-old granddaughter, Léa—who I never would have thought of giving the book to—borrowed a copy. "Sounds interesting!" she told me.

When I shared these reader reactions with François Parpaix, he told me he wasn't surprised: young people are saturated with sex. From the internet and pornographic films, to the constant press articles about orgasms being compulsory or about methods for completion and ejaculation, the constant focus on sex ends up taking all the mystery out of sex. Yet, as we know, desire needs mystery. François kindly told me, "In your book, you help us discover a different kind of sexuality, one that is less hurried, more emotional, and more sensual—freed from the restricting pressures of performance. I think young people need that very perspective."

I took the initiative of asking Marine Uhissy, a young Belgian journalist who—in her own words—belongs to "the Tinder and online-dating generation" if she would write a few lines about what she gained from reading this book. She notes, "It makes me reflect on who I am—a young woman with an energetic body, but whose way of handling sex might be too automatic and repetitive." Marine told me she has grown aware that her body's youthfulness isn't eternal and that "performance" sex won't always be an option. For her, my book teaches how to lay that kind of sex to rest in order to seek out a different kind of sexual fulfilment, one that comes through exploring unknown horizons. And how exciting! That, above anything else, is what piqued her interest, especially in this day and age, when young people still want to know and try everything yet are inspired to (re)turn towards a more authentic and natural lifestyle. After all, how many young "wild sex" aficionados can truly state that they are 100 percent satisfied and fulfilled?

"Desire needs mystery."

Marine pursues this point in her letter: "The thought that sexual happiness is not singularly restricted to coital sex but can equally include intimacy, tenderness, and empathy is not absurd and it isn't just for 'old people.' On the contrary, it's a new challenge, a real mystery, and one that we would like to start studying right away ... Which is what we endeavor, little by little, by taking a look at the diverse themes presented in *Sex After Sixty*, such as the Eastern erotic arts, the *Kamasutra*, Tantra, and orgasmic meditation ... Why must we wait for our bodies to function less fully in order to discover an erotic sex that is more intentional, sensual, and spiritual if it will help us live more fulfilling sexual relationships?"

The second surprise ensued from the number of women who wanted to find out more about Tantra. I was asked whether I would be willing to host workshops on developing sexuality after the age of 60. People are hungry for a different kind of sexuality, more meditative and aware, but the subject is so taboo that these women keep that desire to themselves. When they are in a relationship, they tell me they would like their partner to take part in this sensual dance, which they feel is possible. They suspect they can potentially help their partner overcome the eventual loss of erectile function and explore something else, an erotic communion that is no less satisfying. But they need help. This implicit request in the letters I have received has led me to give it some serious thought and explore the topic further.

Finally, I had a conversation with my friend Jean-Olivier.[116] We were eating one morning at a café near the port on the island of Yeu, off the coast of western France. Having just read *Sex After Sixty*, Jean-Olivier said to me, "There's something missing from your book. You need to talk about love, including sexual love, between two people whose health is failing. The 'pure love' that bonds a man and woman who know they are going to die, people in a state of 'absolute poverty, having nothing else to lose when they will soon lose their life.'" He told me about what he experienced with his wife, Marie-Françoise, in the final weeks of her battle with brain cancer. He had also just been informed that he was sick and that it wouldn't be long before he followed her into death. "We never loved each other as much as we did throughout those last months, when we had nothing left to lean on, besides being there with each other. We experienced what millions of couples have before us, a love that is free." He explains to me that as Marie-Françoise grew increasingly ill, nearing death and no longer able to control her body, she told him she had never loved him more. And the same applies to him: he had never loved her more than then. He asks himself, "Where did this joy interlaced with sorrow come from? This pure love that was so peaceful, so sweet, so strong, while we were so weak?"

I wanted to include this testimony because it bears witness to the strength of love, to love persisting even in the experience of those who have lost nearly everything. What a beautiful conclusion to a book that seeks to show the powerful bonds of love, the joy of love, even when our bodies no longer can.

ACKNOWLEDGEMENTS

• • •

I'D LIKE TO thank Macha Méril, Brigitte Lahaie, Annie de Vivie, Dr François Parpaix, Dr Olivier Soulier, Jean-Louis Terrangle, Éric-Emmanuel Schmitt, Jacques Lucas, and Marisa Ortolan, all my friends, and all the older men and women who agreed to talk to me anonymously about a subject that is very intimate and taboo in our society, and in so doing break down the barrier of silence that prevents us from seeing the truth.

WORKS CITED

• • •

Publications

de Beauvoir, Simone, *L'invitée* (Éditions Flammarion, 1973)

Brunel, Sylvie, *Un escalier vers le paradis* (JC Lattès, 2014)

Chang, Jolan, *The Tao of Love and Sex* (Penguin Compass, 1991)

Châtelet, Noëlle, *Madame George* (Le Seuil, 2013)

Dadoun, Roger, "Manifeste pour une vieillesse ardente"
(Zulma, 2005)

Daedone, Nicole, *Slow Sex: the art and craft of the female orgasm*
(Grand Central Publishing, 2011)

Dall'Aglio, Yann, *Jt'm, l'amour est-il has been?* (Flammarion, 2012)

Ferber, Jacques, *L'amant tantrique* (Le Souffle d'Or, 2007)

Fiat, Éric, "Champagne et tisane. Approche philosophique des
amours de vieillesse," in *Amours de vieillesse* (EHESP Press,
April 2009)

Foenikos, David, *Les souvenirs* (Gallimard, 2011)

Habib, Claude, *Le goût de la vie commune* (Flammarion, 2014)

de Hennezel, Marie, *The Warmth of the Heart Prevents the Body
from Rusting: ageing without growing old* (Scribe, 2012)

Héril, Alain, *Femme épanouie: mieux dans son desire, mieux dans son plaisir* (Payot, 2012)

Jullien, François, *De l'intime: loin du bruyant amour* (Grasset, 2013)

Lahaie, Brigitte, *Le couple et l'amour* (J'ai Lu, 2006)

Larue, Michèle, *Osez ... le sexe tantrique* (La Musardine, 2012)

Lemoine-Darthois, Régine and Weissman, Élisabeth, *Un âge nommé désir* (Albin Michel, 2006)

Long, Barry, *Making Love: sexual love the divine way* (Barry Long Books, 2006)

Malraux, André, *The Royal Way* (Random House, 1961)

Méril, Macha, *Biographie d'un sexe ordinaire* (Albin Michel, 2003)

Méril, Macha, *Si je vous disais* (Albin Michel, 2004)

Misrahi, Robert, *La joie d'amour: pour une érotique du bonheur* (Éditions Autrement, 2014)

Nancy, Jean-Luc and Van Reeth, Adèle, *La jouissance* (Poche, 2014)

Nin, Anaïs, *The Diary of Anaïs Nin, Volume 4 1944–1947* (Harcourt Publishers Ltd, 1980)

Parpaix, François, *Pour être de meilleurs amants* (Robert Laffont, 2004)

Perel, Esther, *Mating in Captivity: sex, lies and domestic bliss* (Hodder & Stoughton, 2007)

Price, Joan, *Better Than I Ever Expected* (Seal Press, 2005)

Simpère, Françoise, *Il n'est jamais trop tard pour aimer plusieurs hommes* (La Martinière, 2003)

Simpère, Françoise, *Ce qui trouble Lola* (Éditions Blanche, 2004)

Terrangle, Jean-Louis, *La caresse de l'ange* (Presses de la Renaissance, 2002)

Tiberghien, Gilles A., *Aimer: une histoire sans fin* (Flammarion, 2013)

Vasey, Stephen, *Laisser faire l'amour: un chemin surprenant vers la lenteur sexuelle* (Love of the Path, 2013)

Vizinczey, Stephen, *In Praise of Older Women* (Penguin Modern Classics, 2010)

Articles/websites

Angot, Michel, *L'art érotique hindou* http://www.clio.fr/bibliotheque/pdf/pdf_lart_erotique_hindou.pdf

Bettencourt, Ricki, Barrett-Connor, Elizabeth, and Trompeter, Susan E., "Sexual activity and satisfaction in healthy community-dwelling older women," in *The American Journal of Medicine* (January 2012)

Desages, Caroline Franc, in *L'Express* (15 September 2014)

Haworth, Abigail, "Why have young people in Japan stopped having sex?," in *The Guardian* (20 October 2013) www.theguardian.com/world/2014/oct/20/young-people-japan-stopped-having-sex

Kraland, Stanislas, "La sexualité des personnes âgées au cœur d'une démarche inédite de formation en maisons de retraite," in *Huffington Post* (19 June 2013)

Loret, Éric, "Le 'ça' et le sexe," in *Libération* (7 August 2014)

Parpaix, François, www.couple-et-sentiments.fr

www.quinquessence.fr

Trudel, G. and Goldfarb, M.R., "The effect of age on sexual repertoire and its concomitant pleasure," in *Sexologies* (October–December 2006)

Films

Virot, Ludovic, *Le sens de l'âge* (2011)

Public talks

"Our dear departed," talk given by Noëlle Châtelet at the Audiens
conference on "Les chemins du deuil" (15 November 2014)

Surveys

"Age and pleasure," Ipsos survey (December 2013)
NORC
Colson (2005)
Montenegro (2004)

NOTES

• • •

1. "Age and Pleasure," Ipsos survey (December 2013).
2. Marie de Hennezel, *The Warmth of the Heart Prevents the Body from Rusting: ageing without growing old* (Scribe, 2012), quoted by the author in a television program broadcast on Arte.
3. Twenty years ago, a survey by NORC (the National Opinion Research Center) found that nearly 30 percent of men and 26.7 percent of women aged over 65 make love less than once a month.
4. A classic of ancient Indian literature, written in the 4th century CE.
5. Michel Angot, *L'art érotique hindou.*
6. Erectile dysfunction affects 34 percent of men aged between 60 and 69, 53 percent between 70 and 79, and 81 percent of the over-80s.
7. Nearly every survey gives the same results: four-fifths of men and three-fifths of women stay sexually active until they are 70. The percentage falls to a third of men and a fifth of women after age 75.
8. Some interesting statistics: a recent telephone survey among

507 French women (aged between 20 and 65) revealed that
a quarter of those questioned experience erection problems
in their partners. But 85 percent said it did not affect their
sexual satisfaction. What upset the women the most wasn't
the absence of penetration (3 percent), it was the lack of
communication (18 percent), lack of compensatory caressing
(17 percent), their partner's anxiety (38 percent), or the
fear that their erectile dysfunction signaled a drop in their
partner's desire (Colson, 2005).

9. Brigitte Lahaie, *Le couple et l'amour* (J'ai Lu, 2006).

10. Ibid.

11. Alain Héril, *Femme épanouie: mieux dans son desire, mieux dans son plaisir* (Payot, 2012).

12. Ibid. (my emphasis).

13. Ibid. (my emphasis).

14. "I no longer screw."

15. Divorce rates in the over-60s have probably doubled over
the past 20 years, and a quarter of 54-to-64-year-olds have
already been separated. One study (Montenegro, 2004) found
that 57 percent of men and 54 percent of women claimed to
have an active sex life after they remarried. There is strong
evidence to suggest the percentage is even higher now.

16. The statistics prove it: men who have sex twice per week after
60 increase their life expectancy by 50 percent, potentially
gaining an extra ten years.

17. Yann Dall'Aglio, *Jt'm, l'amour est-il has been?*
(Flammarion, 2012).

18. Ibid.

19. Ibid.

20. *Psychologies* magazine (February 2012).

21. *Libération* (9 and 10 August 2014).

22. Polyamory is a movement founded by Françoise Simpère in Quebec. It encompasses people who are within a committed relationship but who have agreed to let each other have extra-marital relationships with the full knowledge and consent of everyone involved. Polyamory is therefore consensual by necessity and is governed by a specific code of ethics. It is different from swinging or open relationships.

23. Françoise Simpère, *Il n'est jamais trop tard pour aimer plusieurs hommes* (La Martinière, 2003); *Ce qui trouble Lola* (Éditions Blanche, 2004).

24. Interview on *Doctissimo* site (14 August 2014).

25. Éric-Emmanuel Schmitt is a French-born Belgian dramatist, novelist, and director.

26. Esther Perel, *Mating in Captivity: sex, lies and domestic bliss* (Hodder & Stoughton, 2007).

27. François Jullien, *De l'intime: loin du bruyant amour* (Grasset, 2013).

28. Claude Habib, *Le goût de la vie commune* (Flammarion, 2014).

29. Ibid.

30. Ibid.

31. Ibid.

32. Association Bernard Dutant, Sida et Ressourcement, Maison des Associations La Canebière Marseille.

33. Jean-Louis Terrangle, *La caresse de l'ange* (Presses de la Renaissance, 2002).

34. Éric Loret, "Le 'ça' et le sexe," *Libération* (7 August 2014).

35. Abigail Haworth, "Why have young people in Japan stopped having sex?," in *The Guardian* (20 October 2013).

36. Japan's Institute of Population and Social Security reports that 90 percent of young women believe that staying single is preferable to marriage (ibid.).

37. Thirteen million people live with their parents in Japan, 3 million of whom are over 35 (ibid.).

38. Caroline Franc Desages, in *L'Express* (15 September 2014).

39. Sylvie Brunel, *Un escalier vers le paradis* (J.C. Lattès, 2014).

40. Stephen Vizinczey, *In Praise of Older Women* (Penguin Modern Classics, 2010).

41. Macha Méril is an author and actress. She has starred in French films including *Deep Red* (1975), *Belle de Jour* (1967), and *Une Femme Mariée* (1964).

42. Particularly *Biographie d'un sexe ordinaire* (Albin Michel, 2003).

43. HRT is a controversial treatment. Many gynecologists are discouraging their patients from taking it because of the risk of breast cancer, but others claim the risk is not as high as they say, and point out that the American research responsible for the concerns surrounding HRT was conducted on obese women, which completely changes things.

44. Macha Méril, *Si je vous disais* (Albin Michel, 2004).

45. Jean-Luc Nancy and Adèle Van Reeth, *La jouissance* (Poche, 2014).

46. Régine Lemoine-Darthois and Élisabeth Weissman, *Un âge nommé désir* (Albin Michel, 2006).

47. In Hinduism, Shakti is feminine creative power.

48. Robert Misrahi, *La joie d'amour: pour une érotique du bonheur* (Éditions Autrement, 2014).

49. Misrahi was born on 3 January 1926.

50. This "inventiveness" at the heart of love is superbly discussed by Gilles A. Tiberghien in *Aimer: une histoire sans fin* (Flammarion, 2013).

51. Misrahi, op. cit., preface by Michel Onfray.

52. Ibid.

53. Ibid.

54. Ibid.

55. Ibid.: "The person may suffer more from the other's lack of understanding of them, their values and their creations if he or she remains completely silent. Asymmetry (one talks and the other is silent) increases the distance and separation between them."

56. Discussed earlier, in chapter 2.

57. Misrahi, op. cit.

58. Ibid.

59. Ibid.

60. Ibid.

61. Tantra is a sacred sexual practice. In Tantric philosophy, the path to orgasm is more important than the orgasm itself. Therefore, practitioners do not make love to experience intercourse but to enjoy the pleasure and relaxation that arise from the union and fusion of the couple and the alchemy they create. Intercourse inspired by Tantra tends to delay the moment of orgasm so the couple can derive as much pleasure as possible from their fusion.

62. André Malraux, *The Royal Way* (Random House, 1961).

63. Tantra course run by Marisa Ortolan, www.horizon-tantra. com.

64. As a woman and a man, respectively.

65. In sexual yoga, chakras are energy centers located all the way up the spine. The first chakra corresponds to the coccyx, the second to the sexual organs, the third to the solar plexus, the fourth to the heart, the fifth to the throat, the sixth to the third eye, and the seventh to the crown of the head.

66. Alain Héril, op. cit.

67. Led by teacher Jacques Lucas, www.horizon-tantra.com.

68. Barry Long, *Making Love: sexual love the divine way* (Barry Long Books, 2006).

69. Ibid.

70. Ibid.

71. Ibid.

72. Ibid.

73. Ibid.

74. Sanscrit for "vulva" and "penis."

75. For example, "Laisser Faire l'Amour" courses (in French and English) run by Stephen Vasey in Switzerland, France, and Belgium (www.therapie-de-couple.ch); and "The Making Love Retreat," created and run by Diana and Michael Richardson in Switzerland, and by other couples in other European countries (www.livinglove.com).

76. Stephen Vasey, *Laisser faire l'amour* (Love of the Path, 2013).

77. Jacques Ferber, *L'amant tantrique* (Le Souffle d'Or, 2007).

78. In Greek mythology, Tiresias was a prophet who was turned into a woman for seven years then back into a man again. Tiresias ended an argument between Zeus and Hera about whether men or women experience the most pleasure by telling them that women have nine times more pleasure than men.

79. Jacques Ferber, op. cit.

80. Ibid.

81. Quoted by Michèle Larue in *Osez ... le sexe tantrique* (La Musardine, 2012).

82. Marie de Hennezel, *The Warmth of the Heart Prevents the Body from Rusting*, op. cit.

83. Jolan Chang, *The Tao of Love and Sex* (Penguin Compass, 1991). "A book that men always discover too late and should be slipped onto the bedside table of young adolescents so they can discover sexuality in a less scary light," says Cyril Javary.

84. Jolan Chang, op. cit.

85. Su Nu Ching, *Arts of the Bedroom Chamber*, quoted by Michèle Larue, op. cit.

86. Jolan Chang, op. cit.

87. Ibid.

88. Seventy percent of sexually active women over the age of 60 say they are at least as much, if not more, satisfied than when they were 40 years old.

89. An annual survey conducted by the National Council on Aging among 1,300 American women aged over 60.

90. Joan Price, *Better Than I Ever Expected* (Seal Press, 2005).

91. Ibid.

92. Ibid.

93. Nicole Daedone, *Slow Sex: the art and craft of the female orgasm* (Grand Central Life & Style, 2011).

94. Ibid.

95. David Foenkinos, *Les souvenirs* (Gallimard, 2011).

96. Ricki Bettencourt, Elizabeth Barrett-Connor, and Susan E. Trompeter, "Sexual activity and satisfaction in healthy community-dwelling older women," in *The American Journal of Medicine* (January 2012).

97. G. Trudel and M.R. Goldfarb, "The effect of age on sexual repertoire and its concomitant pleasure," in *Sexologies* (October–December 2006).

98. Yann Dall'Aglio, op. cit.

99. Ibid.

100. Robert Misrahi, op. cit.

101. Marie de Hennezel, *The Warmth of the Heart Prevents the Body from Rusting*, op. cit.

102. Noëlle Châtelet, *Madame George* (Le Seuil, 2013).

103. Ibid.

104. Ibid.

105. Noëlle Châtelet, "Our dear departed," talk given at the Audiens conference on "Les chemins du deuil" ("Paths of Mourning") (15 November 2014).

106. Éric Fiat, "Champagne et tisane. Approche philosophique des amours de vieillesse," in *Amours de vieillesse* (EHESP Press, April 2009).

107. According to geriatrician Françoise Forette, 70 percent of older people in assisted living accommodation suffer from Alzheimer's.

108. Stanislas Kraland, "La sexualité des personnes âgées au coeur d'une démarche inédite de formation en maisons de retraite," in *Huffington Post* (19 June 2013).

109. Quinquessence.fr. The site's online store sells erotic products for people aged 50 to 100 and over, because "if you're above this age your ticket is still valid."

110. A caregiving method developed in France that emphasizes eye contact, touch, and verbal communication to convey respect for patients as human beings.

111. *Friedrich Nietzsche: writings from the late notebooks*, edited by Rüdiger Bittner (Cambridge University Press, 2003), p. 182.

112. Yves Semen, *La théologie du corps* (Éditions du Cerf, 2014).

113. Robert Misrahi, *La joie d'amour*, op. cit (italics my emphasis).

114. Ibid.

115. Ibid.

116. Jean-Olivier Héron is an illustrator, writer, and founder of Gallimard Jeunesse.